CONTENTS

REV: 09162024

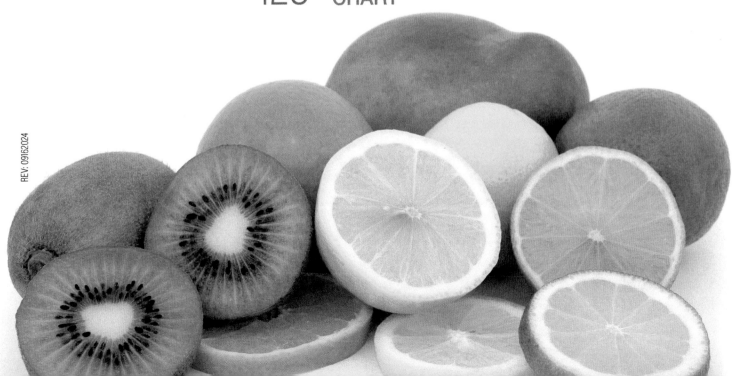

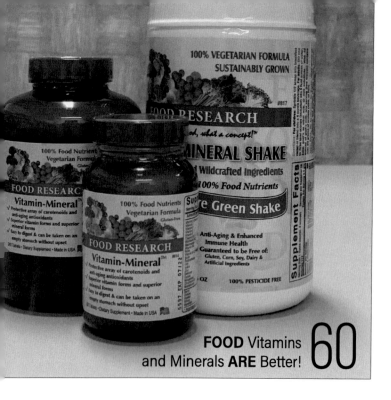

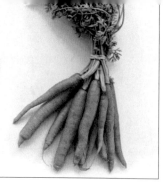

The **TRUTH** About **VITAMINS** in Nutritional Supplements

95

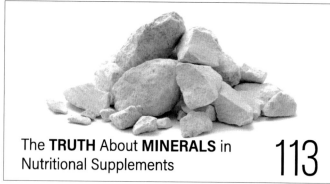

The **TRUTH** About **MINERALS** in Nutritional Supplements

113

FOOD Vitamins and Minerals **ARE** Better! 60

LIST OF ALL FOOD RESEARCH PRODUCTS

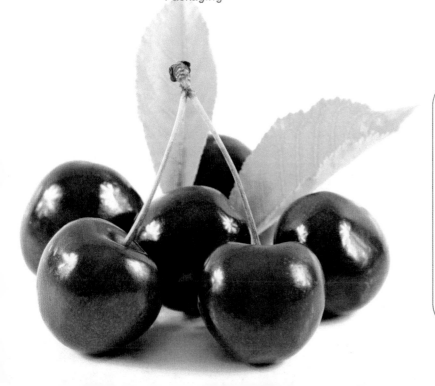

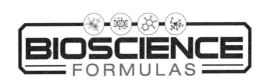

BIOSCIENCE FORMULAS

CALCIUM LACTATE +™

DENTO-GUMS™

LITH-MAG-FORTE™

OUR MISSION

Doctors' Research is dedicated to improving the quality of everyone's life by providing the safest, the best, and the most effective 100% **FOOD** supplements available through health care professionals.

OUR CORPORATE VALUES

Doctors' Research demonstrates its commitment to the world by:

Providing only 100% **FOOD** products from **Food Research International, LLC** to health care professionals.

Never providing any vitamins or mineral from USP or inorganic source in our products.

Utilizing environmentally friendly practices in the growing and processing of the foods that go into the dietary supplements.

Never using porcine, shellfish, or USA-derived bovine in any products.

Never utilizing gelatin for capsules (or anything else).

Publishing in scientific journals the benefits of 100% whole food nutrients and other ingredients in dietary supplements.

Utilizing techniques which have been proven over decades to provide the best quality 100% food dietary supplements.

Having the very best vegan vitamin and mineral-containing 100% food products on the market. While rocks and petroleum derivatives may legally be labled "vegan", they are not 100% food and are not in any **FOOD** brand products.

Having products tested for quality to insure that they exceed the highest standards in the dietary supplement industry.

Never compromising on providing only those forms of vitamins and minerals as found in real foods along with the naturally-occurring health promoting food substances (such as protein-chaperones and enzymes) as dedicated health care professionals expect.

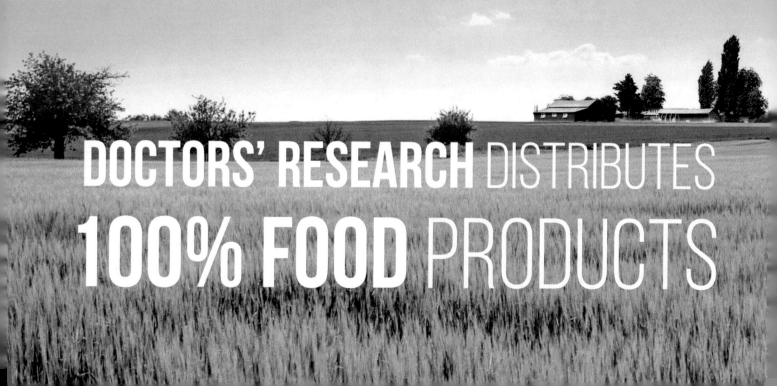

DOCTORS' RESEARCH DISTRIBUTES 100% FOOD PRODUCTS

Don't break the chain!™

FOOD... Doctors' Research is about *Food* - Other nutrient companies are not. All professional supplements distributed by Doctors' Research are 100% *Food!* Our slogans, our processes, and our products are all about *Food.* When we at Doctors' Research say, ***Don't break the chain!,*** we mean don't break the *Food* chain. We are surprised that other supplement companies seem to feel that it is 'natural' for humans to eat synthetic vitamins, most of which are not even the same chemical form (and less of which are in the same structural form) as vitamins found in *Food.* We are surprised that most other supplement companies seem to feel that it is 'natural' to supplement human nutrition with chemically-treated crushed rocks and petroleum derivatives. While nature teaches us that plants have the ability to ingest these types of substances and render them as *Food,* it also teaches us that humans are not plants and should not directly consume crushed rocks.

Humans naturally do not consume soil or other crushed rocks. If they do, medically the condition is termed 'pica' or 'geophagia.' Yet everyday, millions of Westerners (generally unknowingly) consume dozens of industrial processed rocks to 'supplement' their diets--these products normally contain dozens of substances that are not natural for humans to consume. Should people swallow rocks, industrial chemical compounds, petroleum derivatives, ammonia, and cyanide daily? Well, they do. Should your body, or the bodies of your clients, be a dumping ground for these industrial substances? We think not!

We at Doctors' Research understand the need for supplementation, given modern lifestyles and the availability of highly processed foods. However, we feel that supplementation should be from *Foods* and that these *Foods* should contain their nutrients in the same chemical and structural forms as those found in real human *Foods.* We also feel that the supplements should contain the *Food* factors needed for proper absorption and utilization. Even modern science recognizes that minerals need protein chaperones for optimal absorption, yet isolated mineral salts (as are commonly found in so-called 'natural' supplements) do not contain them. *Foods* (including the Foods used at Food Research International Ltd) do naturally contain these substances.

Foods distributed by Doctors' Research are normally specially-grown, with most being hydroponically farmed (since the US has not established organic standards for hydroponically farmed *Foods,* we cannot currently label our US products as

organic). Our growing processes build on the laws of nature, as it is well known that plants will increase their absorption of nutrients if more nutrients are present in their environment. The plants are then harvested, dried under controlled conditions, and put into forms which allow tableting. The *Foods* we commonly use include acerola (cherry), citrus, carrots, herbs (various), kelp, nutritional yeast, mushrooms, rice and rice bran, and spinach. Our *Foods* contain no Genetically Modified Organisms (GMOs), based on average laboratory analysis. In some of our specialty formulas we also include pasture-raised bovine glandulars. Our products do not cause nor contribute to 'yeast-infections' (actually, research suggests that the nutritional yeast we use helps the body combat those types of infections), and the cell wall of our nutritional yeast has also been enzymatically-processed to improve nutrient absorption and decrease the possibility of any food sensitivity.

Because our products are *Food,* it is not necessary to consume them with Food (though they certainly can be). Food ingredients sometimes will vary from those listed in our literature. Many people who previously have complained of problems associated with the commonly sold synthetic, crushed-rock, 'natural' vitamin and mineral formulas, have reported that they have been able to tolerate and benefit from our *Food* products.

Our clinical research group is headed up by Robert Thiel who holds a Ph.D. in Nutrition Science as well as a doctorate in Natural Health. Dr. Thiel authored the world's leading MEDLINE medical journal article on natural vitamins. Dr. Thiel has been named *Research Scientist of the Year* and *Physician of the Year* plus has received the *Orthomolecular Leadership Award* for his leading edge natural health research. He was a licensed naturopathic physician in Idaho and has been a licensed scientist in the State of Alabama since 2003.

Unlike some companies, we do not engage in slick marketing. Our literature contains solid scientific information--we encourage you to read all of it. We believe that since you are interested in truly natural health, you will recognize the benefits associated with using real *Food* supplementation, as well as the benefits of avoiding industrial chemicals that are in other companies' products. We truly appreciate your interest in our products and trust you will share our story with your clients.

- **100% FOOD** Products
- Grown Nutrients With Assays
- HPLC Validated
- Cold Fused and Low Temperature Processed

- **100% FOOD** Nutrients
- Professional Quality Products
- Digestive Disintegration Tested Nutrients
- Nutrients Grown in an FDA Registered Facility

As a health professional, you need to decide whether **FOODS** or industrial chemicals are right for you and your clients.

The FOUR VITAMIN Categories

	SO-CALLED "NATURAL"	SO-CALLED "FOOD BASED"	CULTURED	FOOD VITAMINS
Constituents	So-Called "natural" vitamins are also called USP or pharmaceutical grade.	USP vitamins mixed with some food.	Regular vitamins mixed with food and then cultured.	Vitamins in food. A complete food matrix with protein chaperones.
Structure	Mostly crystalline.	Mostly crystalline.	Uncertain.	Rounded, never crystalline.
Source	Often petroleum derivatives, animal products, and/or hydrogenated sugar.	Often petroleum derivatives, animal products, and/or hydrogenated sugar.	Foods, see below.	Foods, see below.
Type and Quantity of food	No food.	Vitamin value not provided by the added food, but by the synthetic vitamin.	Cultured foods: conceptually like Yogurt, Miso, Sauerkraut. Percentage of food unknown.	Whole "Live" Foods: Carrots, Oranges, Cabbage, etc. 100% Food.
Chemical Form	Usually unnatural.	Usually unnatural.	Unclear.	Natural (as found in Foods).
Nutrient toxicity	Possible, if high amount consumed.	Possible, if high amount consumed.	Not known.	No toxicity associated with vitamins found in plant foods.
Fillers; Binders; Artificial Colors	*Often, Yes.	*Often, Yes.	Uncertain	Rice bran used as a filler/binder. No artificial colors.
Type of Nutrient Delivery	No protein chaperones- Must be found in the body (cannibalization) or a meal.	Potential chaperones found in the added food.	Potential chaperones found in foods.	The protein chaperones are part of the food matrix.
Suggested Use For Maximum Utilization	Must be taken with the right foods. High quality meal helpful for providing nutrient delivery factors for utilization.	Taken any time.	Taken any time.	Taken any time. 100% food with naturally occurring nutrient delivery factors. Ultimate utilization.
This Product is Right For:	Only those who eat high quality meals when taking their tablets and do not prefer real vitamins.	People who don't have the time or knowledge to take their supplements with a quality meal.	Those people who prefer the alterations created in cultured foods.	Everyone who wants the ultimate in nutrient utilization and is interested in real food.
Advantages	Seemingly low price, smaller tablets.	Sometimes increased nutrient utilization than USP vitamins.	Cultured USP vitamins in tablet form.	100% real food. Food is natural for humans.
Disadvantages	No Food. Not in the same chemical/structural form as found in food.	Needs chaperone transformation to be utilized.	Needs chaperone transformation to be utilized.	None known.

The FOUR MINERAL Categories

	SO-CALLED "NATURAL"	LIQUID	CHELATED	FOOD
Constituents	So-Called "natural" minerals are essentially crushed rocks processed with one or more industrial chemicals.	Normally, dissolved rocks.	Element attached to ? (Varies by supplier)	Minerals in food. A complete food matrix with protein chaperones.
Structure	Mostly crystalline.	Varies.	Varies.	Rounded (as that is how minerals naturally exist in Foods).
Chemical Form	Mineral Salts (rocks processed with industrial acids).	Varies.	Varies.	Mineral attached to food factors.
Utilization	Fair.	Fair. Often better than rocks	Fair. Often better than rocks	BEST-optimized by the presence of protein chaperones needed for nutrient delivery.
Nutrient Toxicity	Possible. Body must dispose of "other half" of chemical compound.	Possible.	Possible	Food contains protective factors which help prevent mineral toxicities.
Fillers, Binders, Artificial Colors	Often, yes.	Often, Yes.	Uncertain.	Rice bran used as a filler. No artificial colors/binders
Type of Nutrient Delivery	No protein chaperones- Chaperones must be found in the body or in a meal.	Generally void of chaperones found in foods.	Potential chaperones may exist in chelate.	The protein chaperones are part of the food matrix.
Suggested Use For Maximum Utilization	Must be taken with the right foods. High quality meal needed to provide nutrient delivery factors for utilization.	Taken any time. High quality meal needed to provide nutrient delivery factors for utilization.	Taken any time. High quality meal needed to provide nutrient delivery factors for utilization.	Taken any time. 100% of tablet is food with naturally occurring nutrient delivery factors. Ultimate utilization.
This Product is Right For:	Those that believe eating rocks is fine.	People who don't have the time or knowledge to take their supplements with a quality meal.	Those people who prefer the alterations created in chelated minerals.	Everyone who wants the ultimate in nutrient utilization available only in real food.
Advantages	Seemingly low price-smaller tablets.	Greater nutrient utilization than most rocks.	Chelated meal in tablet form.	100% real food.
Disadvantages	Not food. Not natural for humans. Eating rocks can be a sign of geophagia or pica.	Low potency of many minerals.	Chelated is not a defined term and some chelates are really the same as rock minerals.	None known. Humans have been consuming food since pre-history.

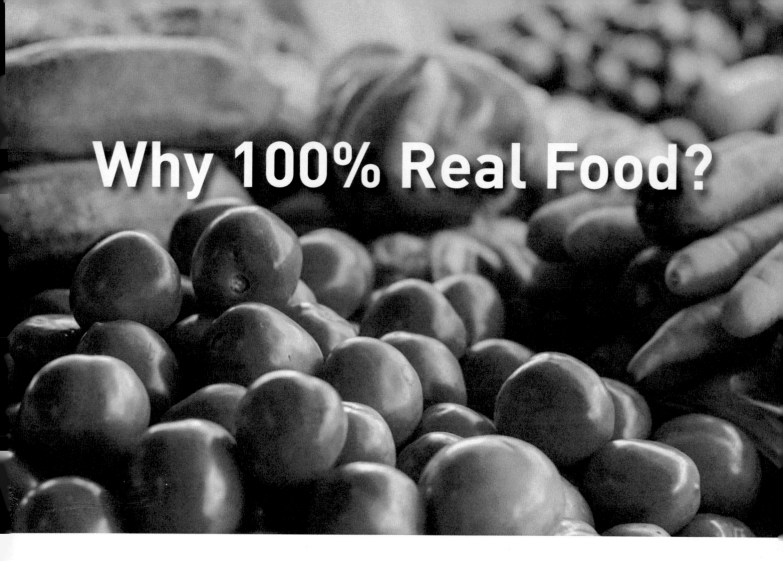

Why 100% Real Food?

Health care professionals with an interest in natural health are aware that many of their patients have nutritional problems with their diets. This is most often due to less whole foods in the food supply, food processing, and sometimes poor dietary choices.

Modern technology has devitalized many foods. According to a US Surgeon General's report, 9 of 10 Americans will die of a disease due to nutrition or lifestyle choices.

This simply should not be.

So, is the solution to this problem consuming vitamins and minerals in isolated USP (United States Pharmacopeia) forms?

We at Doctors' Research think not!

We are sure, as a health professional, you agree that the solution to technologically overly-refined and overly isolated foods is not to base supplementation on USP isolated **"nutrients"** (which are not real food).

Only real foods contain enzymes, protein chaperones, and other substances and co-factors needed for nutrient utilization and transport. There is no reason to give patients inferior formulas that contain isolates that do not include the supporting substances naturally found in foods.

Diet is Important

Dietary choices for your patients are important. Most of them should eat less sweets, hydrogenated fats, refined carbohydrates, and other modern chemically-laden "foods."

While many patients will make some efforts along those lines, as a health professional you know that most may not be willing to make enough changes, either quickly enough or long enough, to promote optimal health.

It is possible that many of your clients are not even aware of what real food supplements are. Hence, there is a real need for 100% food containing dietary supplements.

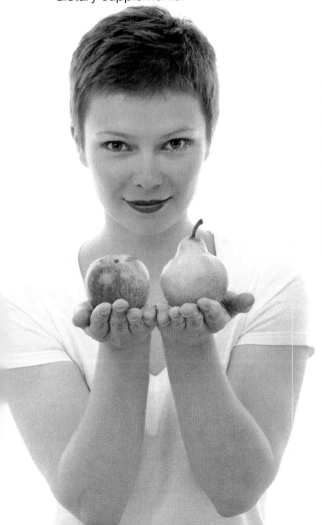

How Can My Patients Know that a Supplement is 100% Food?

Because many companies call their products "**natural**" or somehow imply that they are "**organic**" or "**whole food,**" many of your patients probably believe that is what they are getting.

But unless they are taking **FOOD** brand supplements they probably are consuming isolates (USP vitamins and inorganic mineral salts) which are not food.

In order to tell for sure, it is best to carefully look at the label.

If a supplement product does not state "**100% Food**" on the label, then it is normally safe to conclude that it is not actually 100% food.

There are some words commonly found on many supplement labels that show that the supplement contains USP vitamins and/or inorganic mineral salts.

The most common words to watch out for are:

Ascorbic acid	Thiamin HCL (or thiamin
Calcium carbonate	hydrochloride)
Calcium lactate*	Thiamin mononitrate
Chromium picolinate	Pyridoxine hydrochloride
Cyanocobalamin	Vitamin A acetate
Folic acid	Vitamin A palmitate*
Magnesium oxide	Vitamin E acetate
Niacin	Zinc oxide
Pantothenic acid	

For more details (and a more exhaustive list), please see the sections titled "**The Truth About Minerals in Nutritional Supplements and The Truth About Vitamins in Nutritional Supplements.**"

* Note while this can come from food, it is still an isolate. Mixing foods with these items, as some companies do, does not change their chemical properties. Most companies calling their 'vitamins' as "food-based" or "made with real food," simply use a small amount of food as a 'base' or spray chemical synthetic 'vitamins' on the food. That is similar to what companies do who spray synthetic 'vitamins' on their refined grain cereal products.

Where Do You Get 100% Food Nutrient Supplements?

At Doctors' Research!

While many companies seem to imply that they provide 100% food vitamin and mineral supplements, Doctors' Research is the only company, that we are aware of, that does not use USP vitamins and /or inorganic mineral salts (chelates).

We cater to health care professionals and you have the catalog that FOOD brand products distributes to assist you in deciding which products are best for your patients.

What Makes 100% FOOD Supplements the Best?

Dr. Bernard Jensen, an early 20th century advocate of food-based nutrition, once wrote, "When we take out from foods some certain salt, we are likely to alter the chemicals in those foods. When extracted from food, that certain chemical salt, may even become a poison. Potash by itself is a poison, whether it comes from a food or from the drugstore.

This is also the case with phosphorus. You thereby overtax your system, and your functions must work harder, in order to throw off those inorganic salts or poisons introduced...

The chemical elements that build our body must be in biochemical, life-producing form. They must come to us as food, magnetically, electrically alive, grown from the dust of the earth... When we are lacking any element at all, we are lacking more than one element. There is no one who ever lacked just one element.

We don't have a food that contains only one element, such as a carrot entirely of calcium or sprouts totally made of silicon."

Dr. Royal Lee stated, "The best sources of vitamins and minerals are found in whole foods." Dr. Lee felt it was not honest to use the name 'vitamin C' for ascorbic acid. That term 'should be reserved for the vitamin C COMPLEX'.

Unlike companies who imply that their products are only whole foods, our **FOOD** brand products never contain ascorbic acid or extracted mineral salt nutrients. That is the key to truly natural quality ingredients.

FOOD brand supplements are 100% food as natural doctors of old long advocated.

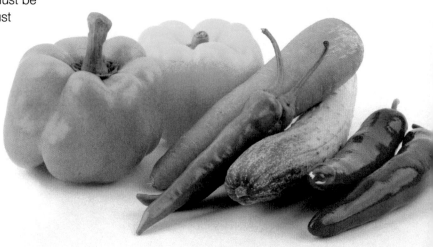

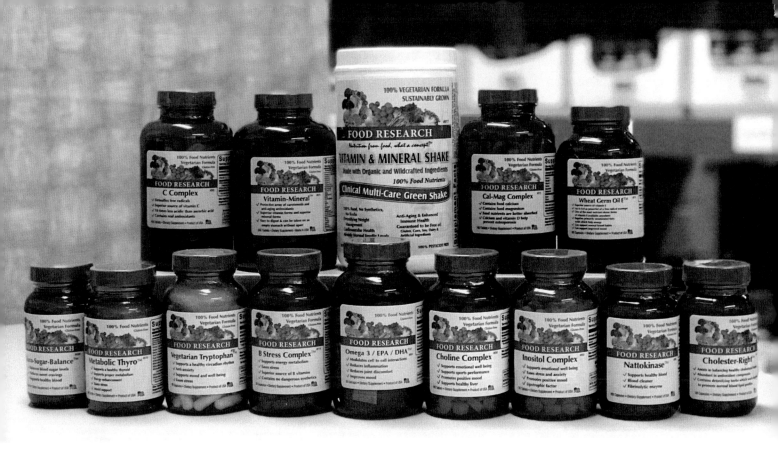

Why are FOOD brand products the best?

At least 98.97% of vitamins consumed are synthetic isolates, though they are often labeled as natural. Yet, there are no isolated USP nutrients that exist naturally. So, nearly all companies `processed minerals in order to produce their vitamin-mineral formulas.

FOOD brand products are different.

> ❝ *At least 98.97% of vitamins consumed are synthetic isolates, though they are often labeled as natural. Yet, there are no isolated USP nutrients that exist naturally.* ❞

They never contain any synthetic/isolated USP nutrients.

FOOD RESEARCH wanted to supply the best possible form of nutrients so it looked into modern technologies that would be compatible with the natural life processes that nature uses to improve the nutrients in natural plants.

In order to obtain the potencies of nutrients that members of modern societies need, many of the nutrients in our products are hydroponically-grown to improve the concentration of nutrients in the specific raw foods that we use.

The processes essentially take advantage of the law of nature that a plant will absorb more of a nutrient when that nutrient is more available. Essentially, the plant is fed an enzyme-containing liquid that will be higher in one particular mineral. The plant will absorb more of that mineral, since more of it is present. The nutrient foods are grown in an FDA registered facility.

In reality this is duplicating the process of nature when we create food nutrients. Nature's process takes inorganic, non-food substances from the soil and delivers them to the cells of the plant. This natural process is the merging of different elements into a union creating one. Creating a whole

11

from different elements is nature in action. The best method of creating a union, like those created by nature, between inorganic fractions and the whole food matrix is achievable through hydroponic technologies.

This led to the acquisition of foods combined with a natural cold fusion process. The definition of fusion is the merging of different elements into a union, creating an enhanced whole from different elements. A natural cold fusion process is used to produce superior nutrients that are always 100% food. Enhanced nutrients occur from the merging of specific elements through a living plant into a whole food matrix through low temperature hydroponic farming.

The reason that the process is "cold" is in order to preserve the naturally-occurring enzymes and other beneficial substances in the foods. Many of the processes and equipment had to be custom-made or altered to accommodate our need to maintain the fresh frozen raw foods used to create the usable raw materials.

Cold fusion processing was not an after thought. No expense was spared to create these cold fusion processes and the state of the art manufacturing plant needed to keep **FOOD RESEARCH INTERNATIONAL, LLC** products the best available on the planet.

Furthermore, this form of **"cold fusion-hydroponic"** farming is pesticide free, and hence the quality of the food nutrients produced this way can be considered superior to conventionally grown foods. After they are grown to proper maturity, the plants are then harvested and dried.

No Genetically-Modified Organisms (GMO) have ever been found in our nutrient foods upon average analysis (which means none have ever been detected any time that our nutrients have been tested for them).

These superior foods are also free of artificial colors, preservatives, and similar chemicals. The grown nutrients are also HPLC (high performance liquid chromatography) validated. The nutrient content of each batch is tested for potency.

FOOD brand supplements represent the best of all worlds: Real food nutrients, in real foods, with naturally occurring substances (such as enzymes,

protein chaperones, amino acids, lipids, and/or bioflavonoids) bottled and tested for potency.

100% food nutrients, 100% of the time.

What Are Glandulars and Why Are FOOD brand Glandulars Better?

Glandulars are animal tissue extracts that have been consumed by humans for thousands of years. In **FOOD** brand products, most of these glandulars have been freeze-dried to ensure that they contain their natural enzymes, peptides, and hormone precursors. **FOOD** brand products only use bovine, ovine, goat, or wild fish for their glandular products.

The source of the bovine glandulars are essentially pasture raised cows from **New Zealand, Argentina and Australia**—USA bovine is never used. Bovine glandulars are often referred to as *cytotrophins,* meaning cell foods. Other bovine glandular extracts are known as *enzomorphogens.*

The oil from the wild herring fish that is in Omega 3/EPA/DHA has been molecularly-distilled for purity to prevent the possibility of toxic metal accumulation.

Does Food Research Have Vegetarian Products?

Yes, we do. At least 37x1 different ones. Vegetarian products are identified by a 'V'.

Food Research vitamins and minerals are from vegetarian sources, they are either wild-crafted or otherwise grown without preservatives, pesticides, fungicides, artificial colors, etc.

Most of the fruits and vegetables listed in the products are organically grown at certified organic farms or wild-crafted. Tests done have found no GMOs (genetically-modified organisms) in any **FOOD** brand products.

Manufacturing Practices

FOOD brand products are produced and/or distributed in three FDA registered facilities. The various manufacturing facilities have passed independent audits to insure compliance with the highest GMP standards.

FOODS are grown, low temperature dried, and slowly ground so they can become part of a capsule or tablet.

The only **"binder"** used for the tablets is purified WATER. The main **"filler"** used for capsules is organic brown rice. Capsules are strictly vegan, except the bovine gelcaps which contain liquids.

To insure the highest possible food integrity, all **FOOD** brand products are made from raw foods. They are processed at low temperatures to retain enzymes and other food components.

This is a difficult standard to meet, so special SLOW processing equipment is often utilized to insure that the products are not processed too quickly as to raise the temperature enough to destroy naturally occurring enzymes and other food constituents.

Wildcrafted and Grown Nutrients

Doctors' Research, Inc. and the various manufacturing facilities used by **FOOD RESEARCH INTERNATIONAL, LLC** are individually US FDA registered facilities.

Many ingredients used in the supplements are organic or wildcrafted and used exactly as they are harvested from nature. However, they are all tested to meet FDA cGMP standards.

Many products have density food nutrient ingredients that have been specially grown. All specially grown nutrients are grown in the United States of America on the East Coast by a company that has been in business since 1977. Prior to the start of the nutrient growing process, the nutrition media must be diluted, clarified, and pH adjusted. This process provides a consistent feed material important for high nutrient growth, that is also free from unwanted microbial contamination or foreign nutrients. Related raw materials are purchased from vendors who meet the strict specifications established for these various materials.

To ensure that the process begins with the best ingredients, each batch of raw material undergoes rigorous scientific testing by the appropriate quality control experts. To guarantee that purity, safety and potency standards for the raw materials, intermediates and finished products are met, each of these materials are subject to sampling, and then quarantined until approval. Once the testing is

completed and approved, a Certificate of Analysis is issued for each individual batch. All manufacturing is based on a lot numbering system, and every batch has a designated lot number for traceability.

The growing process itself begins by adding water to the appropriate food at 95-105°F. The grown nutrients are natural products derived from a pure culture of *Saccharomyces cerevisiae* or other food grown in the proper medium under carefully controlled conditions. Certain nutrients are grown by feeding a controlled amount of the pre-bionutrient embedded into an appropriate glycoprotein to the food during the budding and/or growth process. This controlled metabolization process results in a high bionutrient food product in its most natural environment. Also, during the budding and/or growth process, the pre-bionutrient is added to the budding yeast or re-grown food at an exact concentration, then after a predetermined time the food is harvested. The higher density mineral/vitamin food is then thoroughly washed a number of times with purified water. Then the product, upon enzyme treatment,

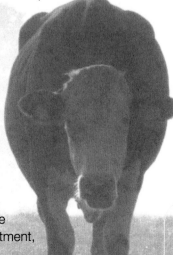

is cold pasteurized, spray-dried and packed. These products provide minerals and vitamins in a form that is readily absorbed and bio-available.

Because the cell wall of the *Saccharomyces cerevisiae* is enzymatically-processed, these nutrients are better tolerated by sensitive people. Also, it does not cause 'yeast infections.' To the contrary the PDR for Herbal Supplements states that *Saccharomyces cerevisiae* is **"antibacterial and stimulates phagocytosis."** In other words, it helps support the immune system. Additonally, Europe's Commission E approved the use of *Saccharomyces cerevisiae* for **"Dyspeptic complaints,"** otherwise known as digestive concerns.

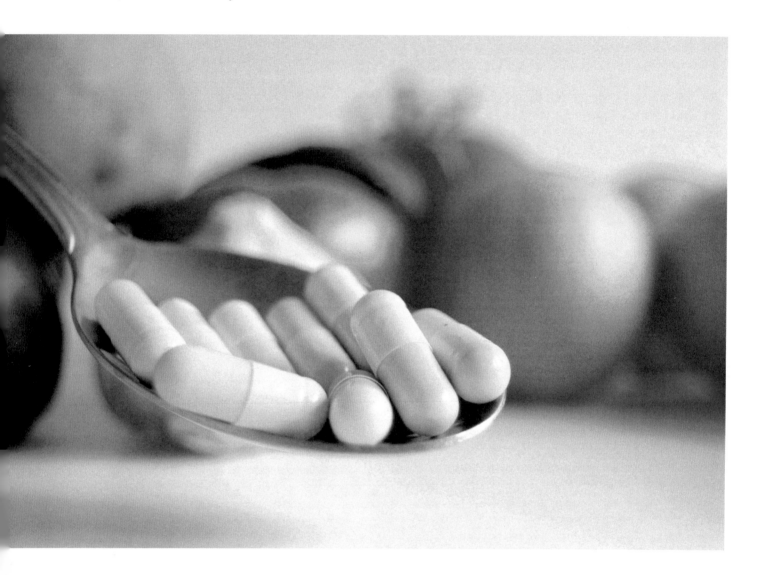

Quality of Food Nutrients

The high nutrient foods are produced using modified OTC drug manufacturing standards. The nutrient growing company has cGMP and GLP protocols in place for the manufacturing of its nutrients. Even though regulations do not require many of these steps, it is believed that by following these strict guidelines, this ensures that the finished product is of superior quality. At the growing facilities, two independent outside contractors are responsible for monitoring water quality and pest control on a monthly and biweekly basis, respectively.

The final high quality products are tested for potency and have been shown to be free of pesticides, herbicides, and heavy metals such as lead.

Quality of the Bottled Food Supplements

All supplements provided are products of the United States of America. The manufacturing facilities are equipped to provide the highest quality nutritional and dietary supplements available. It combines the Food ingredients, bottles, and labels the 100% FOOD nutrient products. All of the manufacturing rooms are temperature controlled, enclosed with full vacuum and particulate collection equipment in place. These techniques ensure quality and avoid cross contamination.

The manufacturing facilities' dedication to superior quality guarantees an extra level of quality assurance. Rigorous quality assurance measures include quarantining all raw materials until composition, identity, and integrity are confirmed and full documentation provided according to the FDA cGMP standards that are observed. The facilities are inspected monthly to ensure cleanliness and safety guidelines are followed. Thorough materials analysis, visual inspection, and laboratory validation ensure only those products that meet the highest standards for purity, potency and efficacy are released for manufacturing and distribution. Only raw materials that meet or exceed specified quality requirements are then purchased. Once the procured material arrives at the facilities they are held until the appropriate quality assurance and quality control teams re-validate the product for identity, purity, and strength.

- **Tablets** are monitored for their size, weight, digestibility, water levels, and integrity. Tableting is done at low enough speeds and temperatures to ensure the integrity of the food components, such as enzymes that the food naturally contains.

- **Capsules** (always vegan) are monitored for their size, weight, digestibility, and water levels. Capsuling is done at low enough speeds and temperatures to ensure the integrity of the food components and that the foods naturally contain.

- **Powders** are monitored for their weight and water levels. Low temperature is used to ensure the integrity of the food components, such as enzymes that the foods naturally contain.

On average, the Food vitamin and mineral products are tested 7-9 times to ensure quality.

Packaging

The majority of **FOOD** brand products are sealed in amber glass bottles. Amber helps protect the food nutrient's from potentially damaging light. Sealing the bottle helps prevent oxidation and helps provide protection from potential product tampering. The glass is recyclable.

All products are bottled/packaged at low enough temperatures to to ensure the integrity of the food components, such as enzymes that the foods naturally contain. We consider that 100% food products are RAW.

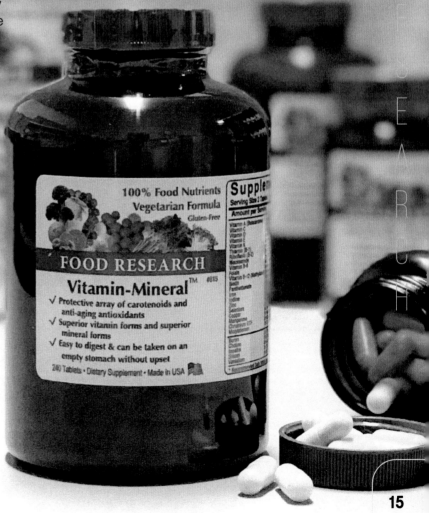

How to Read a Food Research Label

Most companies use synthetic vitamins and/ or acid-processed rocks in their vitamin and mineral formulas. Because ground up rocks exist in nature and the US government has not defined the term 'natural,' many companies attempt to imply that their products are natural by using the term 'natural' when they actually put rocks and petroleum derivatives in their products.

Food Research products are different and include information on labels that help consumers realize that they are different.

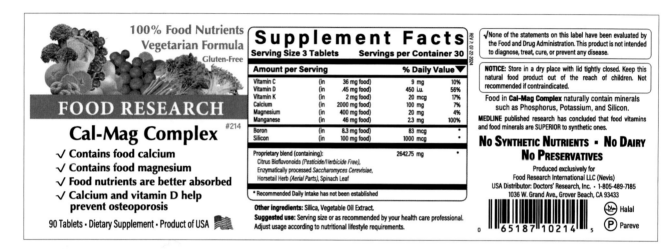

100% Food Nutrients: This means that the vitamins and/or minerals listed on the label are NOT chemical isolates but are part of one or more foods. The individual foods vary, but basically are low-temperature dried foods and contain the natural constituents of foods.

Vegetarian Formula: This means that the product contains no meat. Other than Probio-Zyme-YST, the other vegetarian products are vegan, meaning that they also do not contain any dairy-derived components.

Product Name and Statements: This identifies the product. Below the product name are some statements which provide some information about the product.

Product of the USA: All Food Research products are mixed, formed, and bottled in the USA. The vitamins and minerals show on the label are grown in the USA, with the exception of acerola cherry (which can come from various locations in or out of the USA).

Supplement Facts
(amount of a food and/or a food nutrient are in the product)

- *Information from a typical label on **one vitamin**:*

| **Vitamin C** | **(in 36 mg food)** | **9 mg** | **Daily Value – 10%** |

With this fact, each serving contains 36 mg of a food that is high in Vitamin C which supplies 9 mg of Vitamin C, which is 10% of the Daily Recommended Intake by the US government. Understand that the Daily Recommended Intake by the US government is normally based upon synthetic vitamins or acid-processed rock minerals and may not be the same for those found in food.

- *Information from a typical label on **one mineral**:*

| **Calcium** | **(in 2000 mg food)** | **100 mg** | **Daily Value – 7%** |

With this fact, each serving contains 2000 mg of a food that is high in Calcium which supplies 100 mg of Calcium, which is 7% of the Daily Recommended Intake by the US government.

- *Information from a typical label on one mineral that does not have a **Daily Value %**:*

Boron   **(in 8.3 mg food)**   **83 mcg**   **Daily Value – ***

With this fact, each serving contains 8.3 mg of a food that is high in Boron which supplies 83 mcg (mcg are less than mg) of Boron. The asterisk ('*') shows that there is no specified level Recommended Daily Intake by the US government.

- *Information from a typical label on an **herbal food**:*

Wildcrafted Spinach Leaf   *Spinacia Oleracea*   **30 mg food**   **Daily Value – ***

With this fact, each serving contains 30 mg of a wildcrafted food commonly known as Spinach. The scientific name, *Spinacia oleracea*, is also given. The asterisk ('*') shows that there is no specified level Recommended Daily Intake by the US government.

Other Ingredients
(items involved in the process or coating of the supplement are shown)

- *A typical **tableted** product:*

  Vegetable coating: with this fact, a vegan-source enzymatic coating was sprayed on the finished tablet to aid in swallowing. The coating also makes the tablet stay together better in the bottle to a slight degree. The coating is completely digestible and does not interfere with disintegration and bioavailability during the digestive process.

- *A typical **encapsulated** product:*

  Vegan capsule: with this fact, a vegan-source capsule surrounds the ingredients shown under the **Supplement Facts** box. The vegan capsules that are used have been shown to properly disintegrate during the digestive process.

- *Information on the 'other ingredients' listed in the **Simply Glandular** products.*

  Vegetable Oil Extract helps with the consistency of the product.

  Plant Polysaccharide is a non-GMO corn/rice extract that assists in tableting.

  Silica is a natural substance which helps prevent clumping and aids with uniform distribution of nutrients.

  Digestive Aid is a non-GMO plant cellulose extract that helps the product digest.

Other Information

Suggested use: This is a range of the number of servings typically used. Because **FOOD RESEARCH** products are normally recommended by health care professionals, they may use this as a guideline if they wish.

No Synthetic Nutrients * No Preservatives * No Dairy * Vegetarian: This repeats some of the information elsewhere, but in bold lettering so that it is easier for consumers to notice.

None of these statements on this label have been evaluated by the Food and Drug

Administration. This product is not intended to diagnose, treat, cure, or prevent any disease: When nutritional labels contain statements about the products themselves, these type of 'disclaimers' are required by US laws/regulations.

Doctors' Research, Inc. is a US FDA registered facility and has sent many Food Research labels to the US FDA, but the statements that they have not been evaluated are still required on labels.

Manufacturer and contact information is also on the label as required by US laws/regulations.

Facility certified cGMP by the Natural Products Association: The manufacturer that receives the ingredients, mixes them, encapsulates/tablets them, labels and bottles them is certified cGMP by the Natural Products Association.

Note: Store in a dry place with the lid tightly closed. Keep this natural food product out of the reach of children. Not recommended if contraindicated. Dried food products have a natural attraction towards water, so keeping them in a dry place with the lid tightly closed helps prevent them from absorbing unnecessary liquids. They are recommended to be kept out of the reach of unsupervised children to prevent them from consuming more than they are given. Products are not recommended if contraindicated. Individual circumstances (pregnancy or health conditions), allergies, potential medications, etc. are possible contraindications, and the product should not be taken if it is contraindicated.

Lot number: Products contain a lot number which makes it possible to track. This is required by US laws/regulations.

Most products have a 'BB (Best Before)' date, which is the date by which we expect them to be consumed. The products do not 'expire' then, but some of the nutrients may be less potent after that date. Products distributed are considered to be fresh when sold and then typically consumed.

Superior Bioavailability

While **FOOD** brand labels may be a little more complicated than the typical USP labels, **FOOD** brand nutrients have vastly superior bioavailability.

Ingesting such products as natural food allows the essential nutrients to get to the damaged cells without the body's immune system rejecting them. Food is the best means to deliver appropriate amount of nutrients to the body. However, it has been stated that 75 percent of the American population is deficient in trace minerals. European investigators have also released a report in 2002 revealing that 40 percent of elderly study subjects did not meet daily requirements for iron and calcium.

There are many other valid evaluations that clearly indicate a huge drop in the nutritional values of today's food. Attending to these fundamentals, and the often poorly understood requirements, are a priority consumers need to put at or near the top of their list.

Even as consumers become more interested in the beneficial aspects of nutraceuticals, they are searching for lower doses and easier ways to consume them.

Offering products with the natural targeted delivery systems such as Carrier Food Factors (CFF) increases the usefulness of the products. Natural foods and related targeted delivery technologies are generally designed to deliver measurable amounts of an ingredient to a specific site as well as to improve the efficacy of a product by routing it to where it is needed the most...same principle as in natural food. Foods and 100% food nutrients result in superior bioavailability.

Products are tested to insure that what is on the label is what is in the bottle.

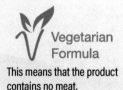
This means that the product contains no meat.

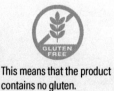
This means that the product contains no gluten.

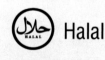
This means that this product is Halal certified.

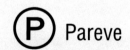
This means that the product contains neither dairy nor meat.

100% FOOD · NO SYNTHETIC NUTRIENTS · NO DAIRY · NO PRESERVATIVES

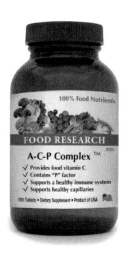

A-C-P Complex™

#125
180 Tablets

√ Provides food vitamin C

√ Contains "P" factor

√ Supports a healthy immune system

√ Supports healthy capillaries

Supplement Facts
Serving Size 1 Tablet   Servings per Container 180

Amount per Serving				% Daily Value ▼	
Vitamin A (Betacarotene)	(in	25 mg food)		375 rae	41%
Vitamin C	(in	120 mg food)		30 mg	33%
Vitamin E	(in	6 mg food)		1.50 mg	10%
Acerola Cherry		*Malpighia Glabra*		120 mg	*
Alfalfa Whole Plant		*Medicago Sativa*		30 mg	*
Bovine Adrenal Cytotrophin				30 mg	*
Bovine Bone Marrow				5 mg	*
Bovine Bone Meal				15 mg	*
Bovine Kidney Cytotrophin				25 mg	*
Buckwheat Grain (Powder)		*Fagopyrum Esculentum*		50 mg	*
Echinacea Purpurea Root		*Echinacea Purpurea*		20 mg	*
Maitake Mushroom		*Grifola Frondosa*		50 mg	*
Organic Brown Rice		*Oryza Sativa*		20 mg	*
Organic Carrot Root		*Daucus Carota*		40 mg	*
Sunflower Lecithin		*Helianthus Annuus*		10 mg	*
Wheat Germ (Defatted)		*Triticum Aestivum*		120 mg	*
Wildcrafted Wheatgrass		*Elymus Trachycaulus*		10 mg	*

* Recommended Daily Intake has not been established

Other ingredients: Croscarmellose Sodium (*Digestive Aid*), Enzymatically processed *Saccharomyces Cerevisiae*, Vegetable Oil Extract, Silica. Contains No Magnesium Stearate.

Suggested use: Serving size or as recommended by your health care professional. Adjust usage according to nutritional lifestyle requirements.

A-C-P Complex™ combines vitamin complex of A and C with the bioflavonoid complex sometimes called Vitamin P. Bioflavonoids support the healthy function of capillaries, connective tissues and the immune system.

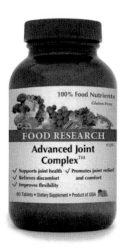

Advanced Joint Complex™

#120 – Small/90T
#123 – Large/270T

√ Supports joint health

√ Relieves discomfort

√ Improves flexibility

√ Promotes joint relief and comfort

Supplement Facts
Serving Size 3 Tablets   Servings per Container 30

Amount per Serving				% Daily Value ▼	
Vitamin C	(in	300 mg food)		75 mg	83%
Vitamin D	(in	.2 mg food)		200 i.u.	25%
Calcium	(in	120 mg food)		6 mg	*
Magnesium	(in	600 mg food)		30 mg	7%
Zinc	(in	30 mg food)		1.5 mg	13%
Boron	(in	75 mg food)		750 mcg	**
Silicon	(in	30 mg food)		300 mcg	**
Acerola Cherry		*Malphigia Glabra*		300 mg	**
Aloe Leaves		*Aloe Vera*		30 mg	**
Bovine Tracheal Cartilage:				300 mg	**
(Chondroitin-Sulfate-A), (Glucosamine/Collagen/Proteoglycan Complex)					
Grape Seed Extract (92+% Proanthocyanidins)				3 mg	**
Organic Alfalfa Leaf		*Medicago Sativa*		63 mg	**
Organic Flaxseeds		*Linum Usitatissimum*		150 mg	**
Wildcrafted Burdock Root		*Arctium Lappa*		300 mg	**
Wildcrafted Cayenne Fruit		*Capsicum Frutescens*		90 mg	**
Wildcrafted Devil's Claw		*Harpagophytum Procumbens*		150 mg	**
Wildcrafted Horsetail		*Equisetum Arvense*		30 mg	**
Wildcrafted Yucca Root		*Yucca Schidigera*		525 mg	**

* Contains less than 2% of the RDI
** Recommended Daily Intake has not been established

Other ingredients: Enzymatically processed *Saccharomyces Cerevisiae*, Vegetable Oil Extract, Silica.

Suggested use: Serving size or as recommended by your health care professional. Adjust usage according to nutritional lifestyle requirements.

Advanced Joint Complex™ is a 100% Food supplement that is intended to supply nutrients, glandulars, and herbs needed to maintain optimal joint health. Bovine tracheal tissue naturally supplies chondrocytes including glucosamine and chondroitin. Herbs, like devil's claw, have long been used to support joint health.

19

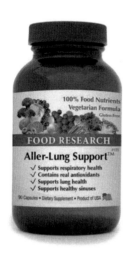

Aller-Lung Support™

#135
90 Capsules

√ Supports respiratory health

√ Contains real antioxidants

√ Supports lung health

√ Supports healthy sinuses

Supplement Facts
Serving Size 1 Capsule   Servings per Container 90

Amount per Serving			% Daily Value ▼	
Vitamin C		(in 48 mg food)	12 mg	13%
Acerola Cherry	Malphighia Glabra		48 mg	*
Bitter Citrus	Citrus Aurantium		77 mg	*
(Naturally Containing Synephrine)				
Bromelain Fruit	Ananas Comosus		40 mg	*
Citrus Bioflavonoid	Quercetin Dihydrate		80 mg	*
Fenugreek	Trigonella Foenum-Graecum		35 mg	*
Organic Brown Rice	Oryza Sativa		10 mg	*
Stinging Nettle Leaves	Urtica Dioica		85 mg	*
Thyme	Thymus Vulgaris		35 mg	*

* Recommended Daily Intake has not been established

Other ingredients: Vegetarian (HPMC) Capsule.

Suggested use: Serving size or as recommended by your health care professional. Adjust usage according to nutritional lifestyle requirements.

Aller-Lung Support™ is a 100% vegan Food supplement that is intended to supply nutrients needed to maintain and support optimal sinus, lung, and immune system health.

Aller-Lung Support™ is only comprised of foods, contains no synthetic USP nutrients or isolated mineral salts, but only contains foods, food complexes, and food concentrates.

 Vegetarian Formula

 Halal   Pareve

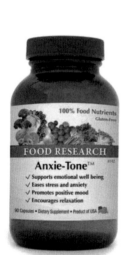

Anxie-Tone™

#142
90 Capsules

√ Supports emotional well being

√ Eases stress

√ Promotes positive mood

√ Encourages relaxation

Supplement Facts
Serving Size 1 Capsule   Servings per Container 90

Amount per Serving			% Daily Value ▼	
Vitamin C	(in	30 mg food)	7.5 mg	8%
Thiamin (Vitamin B-1)	(in	0.7 mg food)	.16 mg	14%
Riboflavin (Vitamin B-2)	(in	2 mg food)	.20 mg	15%
Niacinamide (Vitamin B-3)	(in	4 mg food)	1 mg NE	6%
Vitamin B-6	(in	1 mg food)	.2 mg	11%
Folate (Vitamin B-9)	(in	0.8 mg food)	8 mcg DFE	2%
Vitamin B-12 – Methylated	(in	0.5 mg food)	2.5 mcg	104%
Biotin (Vitamin B-7)	(in	1 mg food)	.5 mcg	1%
Pantothenate (Vitamin B-5)	(in	4 mg food)	1 mg	20%
Choline	(in	12 mg food)	3 mg	*
Inositol	(in	12 mg food)	3 mg	**
Collinsonia Root Powder	Collinsonia Canadensis		100 mg	**
Wildcrafted Passion Flower	Passiflora Incarnata		100 mg	**
Organic Brown Rice Flour	Oryza sativa		44 mg	**
Acerola Cherry	Malpighia Glabra		30 mg	**
Bovine Thymus Cytotrophin			25 mg	**
Bovine Hypothalamus Cytotrophin			15 mg	**
Food Extracted L-Tyrosine (Vegan GMO-Free)			15 mg	**
Wildcrafted Atlantic Kelp	Laminaria Hyperborea		15 mg	**
Wildcrafted Ginkgo Bark	Ginkgo Biloba		15 mg	**
Organic Alfalfa Leaf	Medicago Sativa		2 mg	**
Bovine Parotid Cytotrophin			1 mg	**

* Contains less than 2% of the RDI
** Recommended Daily Intake has not been established

Other ingredients: Enzymatically processed *Saccharomyces Cerevisiae*, Vegetarian (HPMC) Capsule.

Suggested use: Serving size or as recommended by your health care professional. Adjust usage according to nutritional lifestyle requirements.

Anxie-Tone™ is a 100% Food supplement that is intended to supply nutrients, glandulars, and herbs needed for optimal feelings of well-being.

100% Food **Anxie-Tone™** contains vitamin C and many B vitamins, in the forms actually found in reals Foods, which are frequently advised to deal with stress.

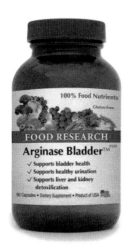

Arginase Bladder™

#160
90 Capsules

√ Supports bladder health

√ Supports healthy urination

√ Supports liver and kidney detoxification

Supplement Facts
Serving Size 1 Capsule   Servings per Container 90

Amount per Serving			% Daily Value ▼
Vitamin C	(in 60 mg food)	15 mg	16%
Acerola Cherry	*Malpighia Glabra*	60 mg	*
Bladderwrack	*Fucus Vesiculosus*	5 mg	*
Bovine Kidney Cytotrophin		20 mg	*
Bovine Liver Cytotrophin		50 mg	*
Buckwheat	*Fagopyrum Esculentum*	50 mg	*
Icelandic Moss	*Cetraria Islandica*	25 mg	*
Organic Beet Root	*Beta Vulgaris*	30 mg	*
Organic Brown Rice	*Oryza Sativa*	8 mg	*
Organic Carrot Root	*Daucus Carota*	30 mg	*
Parsley	*Petroselinum Crispum*	20 mg	*
Rhizopus Oryzae	*Rhizopus Oryzae*	20 mg	*
Wildcrafted Pumpkin Seeds	*Cucurbita Maxima*	20 mg	*

* Recommended Daily Intake has not been established

Other ingredients: Vegetarian (HPMC) Capsule.

Suggested use: Serving size or as recommended by your health care professional. Adjust usage according to nutritional lifestyle requirements.

Arginase Bladder™ is a 100% Food supplement that is intended to supply nutrients to support healthy kidney and bladder function. It also supports the cleansing ability of the kidneys.

The kidneys process proteins and liquids and are the primary organs involved in eliminating metabolic waste products from the blood. Bovine liver naturally contains substances such as the enzyme arginase.

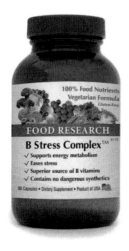

B Stress Complex™

#174
90 Capsules

√ Supports energy metabolism

√ Eases stress

√ Superior source of B vitamins

√ Contains no dangerous synthetics

Supplement Facts
Serving Size 1 Capsule   Servings per Container 90

Amount per Serving			% Daily Value ▼
Thiamin (Vitamin B-1)	(in 24 mg food)	6 mg	480%
Riboflavin (Vitamin B-2)	(in 60 mg food)	6 mg	461%
Niacinamide (Vitamin B-3)	(in 120 mg food)	30 mg NE	187%
Vitamin B-6	(in 33 mg food)	6.6 mg	388%
Folate (Vitamin B-9)	(in 27 mg food)	270 mcg DFE	67%
Vitamin B-12 – Methylated	(in 17 mg food)	85 mcg	3541%
Biotin (Vitamin B-7)	(in 40 mg food)	200 mcg	666%
Pantothenate (Vitamin B-5)	(in 120 mg food)	30 mg	600%
Choline	(in 40 mg food)	10 mg	*
Inositol	(in 40 mg food)	10 mg	**
Organic Brown Rice	*Oryza Sativa*	20 mg	**

* Contains less than 2% of RDI
** Recommended Daily Intake has not been established

Other ingredients: Enzymatically processed *Saccharomyces Cerevisiae*, Vegetarian (HPMC) Capsule.

Suggested use: Serving size or as recommended by your health care professional. Adjust usage according to nutritional lifestyle requirements.

 Vegetarian Formula

 Halal   Ⓟ Pareve

B Stress Complex™ naturally contains carbohydrates, lipids, proteins (including all ten essential amino acids), and superoxide dismutase as found in specially grown, enzymatically processed *Saccharomyces cerevisiae,* and organic brown rice.

Unlike many so-called "natural" formulas, **B Stress Complex™** formula contains no synthetic USP nutrients or isolated mineral salts, but only contains foods, food complexes, and food concentrates.

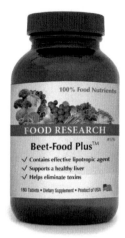

Beet-Food Plus™

#176
180 Tablets

√ Contains effective lipotropic agent

√ Supports a healthy liver

√ Helps eliminate toxins

Supplement Facts
Serving Size 1 Tablet   Servings per Container 180

Amount per Serving				% Daily Value ▼
Vitamin A (Betacarotene)	(in	15 mg food)	225 rae	25%
Vitamin E	(in	9 mg food)	2.25 mg	15%
Vitamin B-6	(in	.85 mg food)	.17 mg	10%
Calcium	(in	10 mg food)	.5 mg	*
Iodine	(in	2 mg food)	30 mcg	20%
Magnesium	(in	10 mg food)	.5 mg	*
Alfalfa Herb			10 mg	**
Bovine Kidney Cytotrophin			10 mg	**
Bovine Liver Cytotrophin			30 mg	**
Bovine Orchic Cytotrophin			10 mg	**
Bovine Prostate Cytotrophin			20 mg	**
Milk Thistle		Silybum Marianum	10 mg	**
Organic Carrot Root		Daucus Carota	65 mg	**
Sunflower Lecithin		Helianthus Annuus	10 mg	**
Wheat Germ (Defatted)		Triticum Aestivum	10 mg	**
Wildcrafted Beet Root		Beta Vulgaris	85 mg	**
Wildcrafted Flaxseeds		Linum Usitatissimum	25 mg	**

* Contains less than 2% of the RDI
** Recommended Daily Intake has not been established

Other ingredients: Croscarmellose Sodium *(Digestive Aid)*, Enzymatically processed *Saccharomyces Cerevisiae*, Vegetable Oil Extract, Silica. Contains No Magnesium Stearate.

Suggested use: Serving size or as recommended by your health care professional. Adjust usage according to nutritional lifestyle requirements.

Beet-Food Plus™ contains beets and beet juice. Beets are a good source of betaine, which has been shown to be an effective lipotropic agent.

Lipotropic agents promote the transportation and use of fats. **Beet-Food Plus™** can sometimes assist with sugar cravings and related issues.

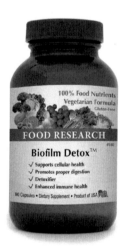

Biofilm Detox™

#180
90 Capsules

√ Supports cellular health

√ Promotes proper digestion

√ Detoxifier

√ Enhanced immune health

Supplement Facts
Serving Size 1 Capsule   Servings per Container 90

Amount per Serving		% Daily Value ▼
Beta-glucanase (Enzyme)	50 BGU	*
Cellulase (Enzyme)	300 CU	*
Endopeptidase (Enzyme)	20000 PPI	*
Exopeptidase (Enzyme)	20000 PPI	*
Glucoamylase (Enzyme)	20 AGU	*
Hemicellulase (Enzyme)	1000 HCU	*
Pectinase (Enzyme)	2500 AJCU	*
Peptidase (Enzyme)	800 HUT	*
Protease with DPPIV (Enzyme)	60000 HUT	*
Serrapeptase (Enzyme)	10 mg	*
Bilberry Berry Extract 4:1	Vaccinium Myrtillus	40 mg	*
Echinacea Purpurea Root	Echinacea Purpurea	25 mg	*
Garlic Bulb	Allium Sativa	25 mg	*
Grapefruit Seed Extract	Citrus x Paradisi	40 mg	*
Milk Thistle Seed	Silybin Marianum	10 mg	*
Wildcrafted Astragalus Root	Astragalus Membranaceus	25 mg	*
Wildcrafted Black Walnut Hull	Juglans Nigra	25 mg	*
Wildcrafted Oregano Leaf	Organum Vulgare	25 mg	*
Wildcrafted Shiitake Mushroom	Lentinula Edodes	25 mg	*

* Recommended Daily Intake has not been established

Other ingredients: Vegetarian (HPMC) Capsule.

Suggested use: Serving size or as recommended by your health care professional. Adjust usage according to nutritional lifestyle requirements.

Biofilm Detox™ is a 100% vegetarian FOOD supplement that supplies herbs and enzymes. These natural substances are intended to help the body rid itself of biofilms that certain pathogenic microorganisms sometimes thrive in.
Biofilm Detox™ naturally contains potassium, carbohydrates, lipids, proteins (including all ten essential amino acids), and protein chaperones as found in the listed foods.

 Vegetarian Formula

 Halal Pareve

22   *Not Recommended During Pregnancy.*

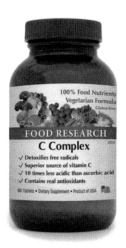

C Complex™

#204 – Small/90T
#205 – Large/270T

√ Detoxifies free radicals

√ Superior source of vitamin C

√ 10 times less acidic than ascorbic acid

√ Contains real antioxidants

Supplement Facts
Serving Size 1 Tablet   Servings per Container 90

Amount per Serving		% Daily Value ▼	
Vitamin C	(in 870 mg food)	217 mg	241%
Acerola Cherry	*Malpighia Glabra*	60 mg	*
Citrus Bioflavonoids	(Pesticide/Herbicide free)	810 mg	*

* Recommended Daily Intake has not been established

Other ingredients: Croscarmellose Sodium *(Digestive Aid),* Vegetable Oil Extract, Silica.

Suggested use: Serving size or as recommended by your health care professional. Adjust usage according to nutritional lifestyle requirements.

C Complex™ is a 100% vegan Food supplement that is intended to supply 100% Food vitamin C. Unlike some other so-called "whole food" vitamins, it does not contain any isolated ascorbic acid. Royal Lee claimed that ascorbic acid was not vitamin C. All the vitamin C in this product comes from oranges and acerola cherries.

C Complex™ has antioxidant abilities. Vitamin C has long been recognized as an important nutrient for supporting cardiovascular, immune, musculoskeletal, endocrine, and other systems.

 Vegetarian Formula

 Halal   Pareve

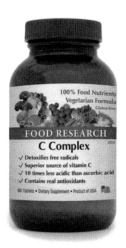

Cal-Mag Complex™

#214 – Small/90T
#215 – Large/270T

√ Contains food calcium

√ Contains food magnesium

√ Food nutrients are better absorbed

√ Calcium and vitamin D help prevent osteoporosis

Supplement Facts
Serving Size 3 Tablets   Servings per Container 30

Amount per Serving			% Daily Value ▼	
Vitamin C	(in	36 mg food)	9 mg	10%
Vitamin D	(in	.45 mg food)	450 i.u.	56%
Vitamin K	(in	2 mg food)	20 mcg	17%
Calcium	(in	2000 mg food)	100 mg	7%
Magnesium	(in	400 mg food)	20 mg	4%
Manganese	(in	46 mg food)	2.3 mg	100%
Boron	(in	8.3 mg food)	83 mcg	*
Silicon	(in	100 mg food)	1000 mcg	*
Citrus Bioflavonoids		(Pesticide/Herbicide free)	36 mg	*
Horsetail Herb (Aerial Parts)		*Equisetum Arvense*	20 mg	*
Spinach Leaf		*Spinacia Oleracea*	30 mg	*

* Recommended Daily Intake has not been established

Other ingredients: Enzymatically processed *Saccharomyces Cerevisiae,* Vegetable Oil Extract, Silica.

Suggested use: Serving size or as recommended by your health care professional. Adjust usage according to nutritional lifestyle requirements.

Food in Cal-Mag Complex naturally contain minerals such as Phosphorus, Potassium, and Silicon.

Cal-Mag Complex™ is a 100% vegan Food supplement that is intended to supply 100% Food minerals and vitamins to support optimal bone health.

It contains naturally occurring carbohydrates, lipids, proteins (including all ten essential amino acids), superoxide dismutase, and truly organic bioflavonoids as found in enzymatically processed *Saccharomyces cerevisiae* and oranges.

 Vegetarian Formula

 Halal   Pareve

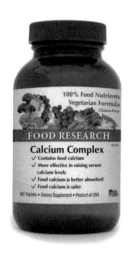

Calcium Complex™

#226 – Small/90T
#227 – Large/270T

√ Contains food calcium

√ More effective in raising serum calcium levels

√ Food calcium is better absorbed

√ Food calcium is safer

Supplement Facts

Serving Size 3 Tablets   Servings per Container 90

Amount per Serving			% Daily Value ▼
Calcium	(in 2610 mg food)	130 mg	10%
Wildcrafted Spinach Leaf	Spinacia Oleracea	100 mg	*

* Recommended Daily Intake has not been established

Other ingredients: Enzymatically processed *Saccharomyces Cerevisiae*, Vegetable Oil Extract, Silica.

Suggested use: Serving size or as recommended by your health care professional. Adjust usage according to nutritional lifestyle requirements.

Vegetarian Formula

Gluten Free

Halal

Ⓟ Pareve

Calcium Complex™ is a 100% vegan Food supplement that is intended to supply 100% Food calcium. Research has shown in groups of people who consume 300 mgs of Food calcium per day or less from plant sources that they have low incidences of osteoporosis.

100% Food **Calcium Complex™** is a plant source of calcium. It does not contain calcium mineral salts such as calcium carbonate, calcium citrate, or calcium lactate.

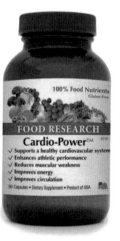

Cardio-Power™

#230
90 Capsules

√ Supports a healthy cardiovascular system

√ Enhances athletic performance

√ Reduces muscular weakness

√ Improves energy

√ Improves circulation

Supplement Facts

Serving Size 1 Capsule   Servings per Container 90

Amount per Serving				% Daily Value ▼
Vitamin C	(in	30 mg food)	7 mg	8%
Vitamin E	(in	21 mg food)	5 i.u.	35%
Vitamin B-6	(in	1 mg food)	.2 mg	11%
Folate (Vitamin B-9)	(in	400 mcg food)	4 mcg DFE	1%
Vitamin B-12 – Methylated	(in	60 mcg food)	.3 mcg	12%
Selenium	(in	4 mg food)	4 mcg	8%
Acerola Cherry	Malphighia Glabra		30 mg	*
Bovine Heart Cytotrophin			193 mg	*
Bovine Liver Cytotrophin			15 mg	*
Garlic	Allium Sativum		15 mcg	*
Organic Brown Rice	Oryza Sativa		26 mg	*
Wildcrafted Hawthorn Berry	Crataegus Monogyna		50 mg	*

* Recommended Daily Intake has not been established

Other ingredients: Enzymatically processed *Saccharomyces Cerevisiae*, Organic Brown Rice, Vegetarian (HPMC) Capsule.

Suggested use: Serving size or as recommended by your health care professional. Adjust usage according to nutritional lifestyle requirements.

Gluten Free

Cardio Power™ is a 100% Food supplement that is intended to supply nutrients, glandulars, and herbs needed to maintain and support optimal cardiac muscle health.

Cardio Power™ also naturally contains carbohydrates, lipids, proteins (including all ten essential amino acids), and truly organic bioflavonoids as found in specially grown, enzymatically processed Saccharomyces cerevisiae. The bovine heart tissue naturally contains vital heart nutrients like co-enzyme Q10.

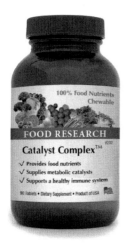

Catalyst Complex™

#232
90 Tablets – Chewable

√ Provides food nutrients

√ Supplies metabolic Catalysts

√ Supports a healthy immune system

Catalyst Complex™ is a multi-vitamin, multi-mineral, trace mineral, and enzyme containing formula. It is a low-dose approach to nutritional supplementation.

Catalyst Complex™ is intended to provide a nutritional Catalyst to promote healthy metabolism.

Supplement Facts
Serving Size 3 Tablets   Servings per Container 30

Amount per Serving				% Daily Value ▼
Vitamin A as Betacarotene	(in	25 mg of food)	375 rae	41%
Vitamin C	(in	360 mg of food)	90 mg	100%
Vitamin D	(in	.5 mg of food)	500 i.u	62%
Thiamin (Vitamin B-1)	(in	1 mg of food)	.24 mg	20%
Riboflavin (Vitamin B-2)	(in	2 mg of food)	.20 mg	15%
Vitamin B-6	(in	4.5 mg of food)	.90 mg	52%
Calcium	(in	25 mg of food)	3 mg	*
Magnesium	(in	40 mg of food)	5 mg	*
Acerola Cherry	Malpighia Glabra		360 mg	**
Alfalfa Juice (Dried)	Medicago Sativa		20 mg	**
Biogurt (Lactobacillus Bulgaricus)			65 mg	**
Bovine Adrenal Cytotrophin			60 mg	**
Bovine Bone Meal			40 mg	**
Bovine Kidney Cytotrophin			40 mg	**
Bovine Liver Cytotrophin			60 mg	**
Bovine Spleen Cytotrophin			60 mg	**
Monkfruit	Siraitia Grosvenorii		900 mg	**
Natural Grape Flavor (Powder)	Vitis Vinifera		450 mg	**
Organic Brown Rice	Oryza Sativa		50 mg	**
Organic Carrot Root	Daucus Carota		40 mg	**
Organic Mushroom Blend	(Cordyceps, Shiitake, Maitaki)		60 mg	**
Organic Strawberry (Powder)	Fragaria × Ananassa		900 mg	**
Organic Sunflower Lecithin	Helianthus Annuus		20 mg	**
Wheat Germ (Defatted)	Triticum Aestivum		100 mg	**
Wildcrafted Parsley Leaf	(Full Spectrum Extract)		60 mg	**
Wildcrafted Wheatgrass	Elymus Trachycaulus		40 mg	**

* Contains less than 2% of the RDI   ** Recommended Daily Intake has not been established

Other ingredients: Enzymatically processed *Saccharomyces Cerevisiae*, Vegetable Oil Extract, Plant Polysaccharide, Silica, Digestive Aid. Contains No Magnesium Stearate

Suggested use: Serving size or as recommended by your health care professional. Adjust usage according to nutritional lifestyle requirements.

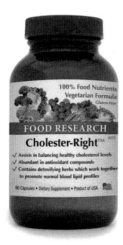

Cholester-Right™

#233
90 Capsules

√ Assists in balancing healthy cholesterol levels

√ Abundant in antioxidant compounds

√ Contains detoxifying herbs which work together to promote normal blood lipid profiles

Cholester-Right™ is a 100% vegan Food supplement intended to nutritionally support the body in balancing healthy cholesterol levels.

Unlike many so-called "natural" formulas, **Cholester-Right™** consists of only foods or food extracts, food complexes, and food concentrates. It does NOT contain any synthetic USP nutrients or isolated mineral salts.

Supplement Facts
Serving Size 1 Capsule   Servings per Container 90

Amount per Serving			% Daily Value ▼
Vitamin C	(in 60 mg food)	15 mg	16%
Acerola Cherry	Malpighia Glabra	60 mg	*
Apple Pectin (Fiber)	Malus Domestica	15 mg	*
Food Extracted Guggul Gum	Commiphora Mukul	110 mg	*
Food Extracted Beta Glucan	Avena Sativa	50 mg	*
Food Extracted Policosanol	Saccharum Officinalis	10 mg	*
Garlic	Allium Sativa	50 mg	*
Organic Brown Rice	Oryza Sativa	23 mg	*
Wildcrafted Atlantic Kelp	Laminaria Hyperborea	10 mg	*
Wildcrafted Ginger Root	Zingiber Officinalis	6 mg	*
Wildcrafted Hawthorn Berry	Crataegus Monogyna	6 mg	*
Wildcrafted Pomegranate Fruit	Punica Gratam	50 mg	*
Wildcrafted Turmeric Root	Curcuma Domestica	5 mg	*

* Recommended Daily Intake has not been established

Other ingredients: Vegetarian (HPMC) Capsule.

Suggested use: Serving size or as recommended by your health care professional. Adjust usage according to nutritional lifestyle requirements.

 Vegetarian Formula

 Halal   Pareve

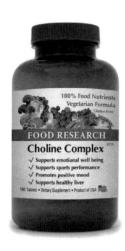

Choline Complex™

#235

180 Tablets

√ Supports emotional well-being

√ Supports sports performance

√ Promotes positive mood

√ Supports healthy liver

Other ingredients: Enzymatically processed *Saccharomyces Cerevisiae*, Vegetable Oil Extract, Silica, Vegetarian Coating.

Suggested use: Serving size or as recommended by your health care professional. Adjust usage according to nutritional lifestyle requirements.

Choline Complex™ is a 100% vegetarian Food supplement that is intended to supply real food choline. Choline is needed to form the neurotransmitter acetylcholine and is also a lipotropic factor.

Choline has been considered as a type of B vitamin. It is required to make phospholipids and other substances necessary for all cell membranes, including myelin sheath which covers nerve cells. It is necessary for gall bladder regulation, liver detoxification, carnitine metabolism, and nerve support.

 Vegetarian Formula

 Halal

 Pareve

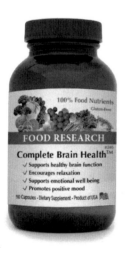

Complete Brain Health™

#245

90 Capsules

√ Supports healthy brain function

√ Encourages relaxation

√ Supports emotional well being

√ Promotes positive mood

Other ingredients: Enzymatically processed *Saccharomyces Cerevisiae*, Organic Brown Rice, Vegetarian (HPMC) Capsule.

Suggested use: Serving size or as recommended by your health care professional. Adjust usage according to nutritional lifestyle requirements.

The brain is the master organ of the body and directly or indirectly controls nearly all processes in the body including movement, intellect, memory, and mood. Bovine brain tissue naturally contains substances such as phosphatidylserine.

Complete Brain Health™ is a 100% Food supplement that is intended to supply nutrients, glandulars, and herbs needed for optimal brain health. It contains pituitary, medulla, and other bovine tissues, along with the antioxidants selenium and vitamin E. **Complete Brain Health™** also contains ribonucleic acid.

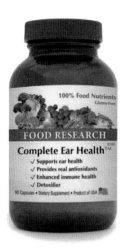

Complete
Ear Health™

#249
90 Capsules

√ Supports ear health

√ Provides real antioxidants

√ Enhanced immune health

√ Detoxifier

Supplement Facts
Serving Size 1 Capsule   Servings per Container 90

Amount per Serving			% Daily Value ▼
Vitamin C	(in 48 mg food)	12 mg	13%
Zinc	(in 15 mg food)	750 mcg	6%
Acerola Cherry	Malphighia Glabra	48 mg	*
Bovine Thymus Cytotrophin		10 mg	*
Chinese Thoroughwax	Bupleurum Chinense	20 mg	*
Food Extracted Co-Enzyme Q10	(Plant Source)	250 mcg	*
Food Extracted N-Acetyl-L-Cysteine	(Plant Source)	10 mg	*
Ginkgo Bark	Ginkgo Biloba	30 mg	*
Wild Caught Cod	(Includes Head and Ears)	21 mg	*
Wildcrafted Icelandic Moss	Cetraria Islandica	161 mg	*

*Recommended Daily Intake has not been established

Other ingredients: Enzymatically processed *Saccharomyces Cerevisiae*, Vegetarian (HPMC) Capsule.

Suggested use: Serving size or as recommended by your health care professional. Adjust usage according to nutritional lifestyle requirements.

Your hearing is important. Hearing problems are exceptionally common. From tinnitus to actually hearing loss, there are numerous hearing problems.

Complete Ear Health™ is a 100% Food supplement that is intended to supply nutrients, glandulars, and herbs needed to maintain and support optimal ear health. Specific glandular tissue naturally contains nutrients needed for the ears. Tillandsia is a type of moss that provides nutrients and has strong absorptive properties.

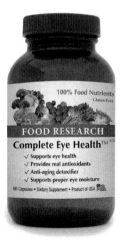

Complete
Eye Health™

#255
90 Capsules

√ Supports eye health

√ Provides real antioxidants

√ Anti-aging detoxifier

√ Supports proper eye moisture

Supplement Facts
Serving Size 1 Capsule   Servings per Container 90

Amount per Serving			% Daily Value ▼
Vitamin A (Betacarotene)	(in 15 mg food)	225 rae	25%
Vitamin C	(in 60 mg food)	15 mg	16%
Vitamin E	(in 2 mg food)	2 i.u.	13%
Zinc	(in 9 mg food)	450 mcg	4%
Selenium	(in 18 mg food)	1.8 mcg	3%
Acerola Cherry	Malphighia Glabra	60 mg	*
Bilberry Berry Extract 4:1	Vaccinium Myrtillus	15 mg	*
Bovine Trachea Cytotrophin		10 mg	*
Eyebright Extract 4:1	Euphrasia Officinalis	20 mg	*
Food Concentrated Lutein	(in 20 mg Marigolds)	1 mg	*
Food Concentrated Zeaxanthin	(in 10 mg Marigolds)	500 mcg	*
Ginkgo Leaf	Ginkgo Biloba	10 mg	*
Organic Brown Rice	Oryza Sativa	5 mg	*
Organic Carrot Root	Daucus Carota	20 mg	*
Wild Cod Liver Oil (Powdered)		20 mg	*
Wildcrafted Broccoli	Brassica Oleracea	10 mg	*
Wildcrafted Rosemary	Rosemarinus Officinalis	20 mg	*
Wildcrafted Tomato Powder	Lycopersicum Esculentum	22 mg	*
Wildcrafted Wolfberries	Lycium Barbarum	40 mg	*

*Recommended Daily Intake has not been established

Other ingredients: Enzymatically processed *Saccharomyces Cerevisiae*, Vegetarian (HPMC) Capsule, Wild Caught Carp (Includes Head & Eyes).

Suggested use: Serving size or as recommended by your health care professional. Adjust usage according to nutritional lifestyle requirements.

Complete Eye Health™ is a 100% Food supplement that is intended to supply nutrients, glandulars, and herbs needed to maintain and support the healthy functioning of the eyes.

Complete Eye Health™ also naturally contains carbohydrates, lipids, proteins (including all ten essential amino acids), and truly organic bioflavonoids as found in specially grown, enzymatically processed Saccharomyces cervisiae and vegetable oils.

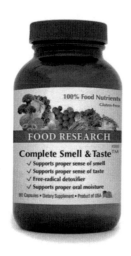

Complete Smell & Taste™

#260
90 Capsules

√ Supports proper sense of smell

√ Supports proper sense of taste

√ Free-radical detoxifier

√ Supports proper oral moisture

Supplement Facts
Serving Size 1 Capsule Servings per Container 90

Amount per Serving			% Daily Value ▼	
Magnesium	(in	212 mg food)	10 mg	2%
Zinc	(in	90 mg food)	4.5 mg	40%
Bovine Liver Cytotrophin			20 mg	*
Bovine Parotid Cytotrophin			2 mg	*
Goat Tongue Cytotrophin			65 mg	*
Wild Caught Cod (Includes Smell and Taste Glands)			11 mg	*

* Recommended Daily Intake has not been established

Other ingredients: Enzymatically processed *Saccharomyces Cerevisiae*, Vegetarian (HPMC) Capsule.

Suggested use: Serving size or as recommended by your health care professional. Adjust usage according to nutritional lifestyle requirements.

Complete Smell & Taste™ is a 100% Food supplement that is intended to supply nutrients, glandulars, and herbs needed to maintain and support optimal olfactory and tongue health.

Complete Smell & Taste™ contains goat tongue and olfactory tissues which contain proteins and other nutrients found in properly functioning taste and smell receptors. Parotid glands support the salivary process and the health of the glands.

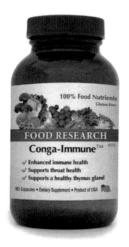

Conga-Immune™

#270
90 Capsules

√ Enhanced immune health

√ Supports throat health

√ Supports a healthy thymus gland

Supplement Facts
Serving Size 2 Capsules Servings per Container 45

Amount per Serving			% Daily Value ▼	
Vitamin C	(in	60 mg food)	15 mg	16%
Zinc	(in	100 mg food)	5 mg	45%
Acerola Cherry	*Malphighia Glabra*		60 mg	*
Alfalfa Leaf	*Medicago Sativa*		20 mg	*
Bovine Bone Marrow Cytotrophin			30 mg	*
Bovine Liver Cytotrophin			50 mg	*
Bovine Lymph Cytotrophin			30 mg	*
Bovine Spleen Cytotrophin			20 mg	*
Bovine Thymus Cytotrophin			100 mg	*
Buckwheat	*Fagopyrum Esculentum*		100 mg	*
Echinacea Purpurea Root	*Echinacea Purpurea*		20 mg	*
Garlic	*Allium Sativa*		20 mg	*
Organic Brown Rice	*Oryza Sativa*		30 mg	*
Organic Carrot Root	*Daucus Carota*		100 mg	*
Organic Shiitake Mushroom	*Lentinula Edodes*		30 mg	*

* Recommended Daily Intake has not been established

Other ingredients: Enzymatically processed *Saccharomyces Cerevisiae*, Vegetarian (HPMC) Capsule.

Suggested use: Serving size or as recommended by your health care professional. Adjust usage according to nutritional lifestyle requirements.

Conga-Immune™ is a 100% Food supplement that is intended to supply nutrients needed to maintain and support optimal thymus, throat, and immune system health. It contains Acerola cherry which is one of the most vitamin C dense foods.

Bovine bone marrow produces B-lymphocytes which are the basis of much of what most consider to be part of the immune system. Bovine thymus tissue helps maintain the thymus gland in a good state of repair to support healthy thymus function.

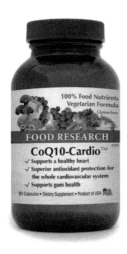

CoQ10-Cardio™

#250
90 Capsules

√ Supports a healthy heart

√ Superior antioxidant protection for the whole cardiovascular system

√ Supports gum health

Supplement Facts
Serving Size 1 Capsule   Servings per Container 90

Amount per Serving			% Daily Value▼
Vitamin C	(in 72 mg food)	18 mg	20%
Acerola Cherry	Malpighia Glabra	72 mg	•
CoEnzyme Q10	(Plant Source)	20 mg	•
Garlic	Allium Sativa	100 mg	•
Organic Brown Rice	Oryza Sativa	8 mg	•
Wildcrafted Hawthorn Berry	Crataegus Monogyna	100 mg	•

* Recommended Daily Intake has not been established

Other ingredients: Vegetarian (HPMC) Capsule.

Suggested use: Serving size or as recommended by your health care professional. Adjust usage according to nutritional lifestyle requirements.

CoQ10-Cardio™ is a 100% vegan Food supplement that is intended to supply nutrients needed to maintain and support optimal cardiac muscle health. CoQ10-Cardio™ supplies plant-source co-enzyme Q10, a nutrient that is important for healthy cardiovascular system function, along with other herbs.

CoQ10-Cardio™ provides nutritional support for the heart, gums, and for overall circulation. It can nutritionally help support the heart, increase endurance, aid with energy, aid with gum health, and promote better overall health.

 Vegetarian Formula   GLUTEN FREE

 Halal   Ⓟ Pareve

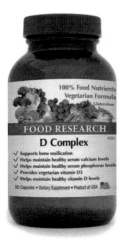

D Complex™

#281
90 Capsules

√ Supports bone ossification

√ Helps maintain healthy serum calcium levels

√ Helps maintain healthy serum phosphorus levels

√ Provides vegetarian vitamin D3

√ D2 naturally present in shiitake mushrooms.

Supplement Facts
Serving Size 1 capsule   Servings per container 90

Amount per Serving		% Daily Value▼
Vitamin D3	(in 5 mg food)	5000 i.u. 625%
Shiitake Mushrooms	Lentinula Edodes	380 mg •

* Recommended Daily Intake has not been established

Other ingredients: Enzymatically Processed *Saccharomyces Cerevisiae*, Vegetarian (HPMC) Capsule.

Suggested use: Serving size or as recommended by your health care professional. Adjust usage according to nutritional lifestyle requirements.

D Complex™ is a 100% vegan Food supplement that is intended to supply 100% Food vitamin D. Vitamin D helps with the absorption of food calcium and even has hormone-like functions within the human body.

Vitamin D helps maintain serum calcium and phosphorus concentrations in a range that supports cellular processes, neurological function, and bone ossification.

 Vegetarian Formula   GLUTEN FREE

 Halal   Ⓟ Pareve

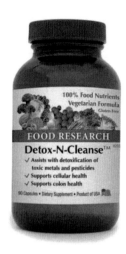

Detox-N-Cleanse™

#285
90 Capsules

√ Assists with detoxification of toxic metals and pesticides

√ Supports cellular health

√ Supports colon health

Supplement Facts
Serving Size 1 Capsule   Servings per Container 90

Amount per Serving			% Daily Value ▼	
Vitamin C	(in 100 mg food)		25 mg	27%
Acerola Cherry	Malpighia Glabra	100 mg	•	
Apple Pectin	Malus Domestica	25 mg	•	
Chlorella	Chlorella Vulgaris	50 mg	•	
Cilantro Leaf	Coriandrum Sativum	15 mg	•	
Collinsonia Root	Collinsonia Canadensis	15 mg	•	
Garlic	Allium Sativa	20 mg	•	
Modified Citrus Pectin		100 mg	•	
Sesame Seed	Sesamum Indicum	35 mg	•	
Slippery Elm	Ulmus Rubra	15 mg	•	
Wildcrafted Wheatgrass	Triticum Aestivum	25 mg	•	

* Recommended Daily Intake has not been established

Other ingredients: Vegetarian (HPMC) Capsule.

Suggested use: Serving size or as recommended by your health care professional. Adjust usage according to nutritional lifestyle requirements.

The outside air is polluted, the indoor air is polluted, water is polluted, and the industrialized food supply is polluted with toxins. Pollution can be a serious issue, so many naturally-minded individuals are justifiably concerned about detoxification.

Detox-N-Cleanse™ is a synergestic blend of foods and food extracts intended to help support healthy colon, urinary system, metal detoxification as well as other detoxification.

 Vegetarian Formula

 Halal   Pareve

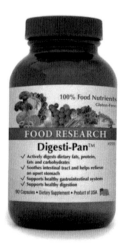

Digesti-Pan™

#295
90 Capsules

√ Actively digest dietary fats, protein and carbohydrates

√ Soothes intestinal tract and helps relieve an upset stomach

√ Supports healthy gastrointestinal system

√ Supports healthy digestion

Supplement Facts
Serving Size 1 Capsule   Servings per Container 90

Amount per Serving			% Daily Value ▼
Amylase		2000 DU	•
Betaine HCL		50 mg	•
Glucoamylase		2 AG	•
Invertase		.05 IAU	•
Lactase		200 LACU	•
Lipase		40 HUT	•
Pepsin		20 mg	•
Protease		5000 HUT	•
Bovine Pancreas Cytotrophin		100 mg	•
Bovine Spleen Cytotrophin		20 mg	•
Ginger Root	Zingiber Officinale	30 mg	•
Okra (Fruit)	Abelmoschus Esculentus	30 mg	•
Wildcrafted Beet Root	Beta Vulgaris	50 mg	•

* Recommended Daily Intake has not been established

Other ingredients: Vegetarian (HPMC) Capsule..

Suggested use: Serving size or as recommended by your health care professional. Adjust usage according to nutritional lifestyle requirements.

Digesti-Pan™ is a 100% Food supplement that is intended to supply enzymes, glandulars, and herbs needed to maintain and support optimal digestive health.

Digesti-Pan™ contains digestive enzymes, pancreatic tissue, betaine hydrochloride, okra fruit, and other herbs. Balance and harmony are important to the entire digestive process because, remarkably, insufficient enzymes can also contribute to constipation and insufficient enzymes can contribute to diarrhea.

Dual Vitality™

#297
90 Capsules

√ Energy and vitality support

√ Supports endurance

√ Supports healthy mood and nervous system

√ Excellent source of beta glucans

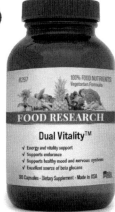

Supplement Facts
Serving Size 2 Capsules   Servings per Container 45

Amount per Serving			% Daily Value ▼
Organic Cordyceps	Cordyceps Militaris	500 mg	*
Standardized beta 1,3 and 1,6 beta glucans			
American Ginseng	Panax Quinquefolius L	400 mg	*
Standardized to 5% [20 mg] ginsenosides			

* Recommended Daily Intake has not been established

Other ingredients: Vegetarian (HPMC) Capsule.

Suggested use: Serving size or as recommended by your health care professional. Adjust usage according to nutritional lifestyle requirements.

 Vegetarian Formula   Gluten Free

 Halal   Ⓟ Pareve

Dual Support for Energy, Vitality, and a Healthy Immune System.

Cordyceps are a type of mushroom. As in all mushroom containing supplements from Food Research, the cordyceps in **Dual Vitality** is supplied by Nammex, the company considered to be the top of the line for supplying the best quality mushroom products to health professionals. "The roots of American ginseng *(Panax quinquefolius)*, contain steroidal saponins called ginsenosides that are purported to be adaptogens (i.e., to increase endurance and improve memory)". Ginseng can protect DNA and help mood.

Feminine Advantage™

#330
90 Capsules

√ Supports female health

√ Enhances mood

√ Supports emotional well-being

√ Helps maintain normal moisture

Supplement Facts
Serving Size 1 Capsule   Servings per Container 90

Amount per Serving		% Daily Value ▼
Black Cohosh	Cimicifuga Racemosa	50 mg	*
Bovine Ovary Cytotrophin		20 mg	*
Bovine Uterus Cytotrophin		50 mg	*
Chaste Tree Berries	Vitex Agnus-Castus	100 mg	*
Mexican Wild Yam Root	Dioscorea Villosa	200 mg	*
Organic Flaxseeds	Linum Usitatissimum	30 mg	*
Red Clover	Trifolium Pratense	50 mg	*

* Recommended Daily Intake has not been established

Other ingredients: Vegetarian (HPMC) Capsule.

Suggested use: Serving size or as recommended by your health care professional. Adjust usage according to nutritional lifestyle requirements.

Once beginning menstruation, a woman's hormone levels change several times per month. As a woman continues to mature, she tends to have different hormonal levels at different times, and even various stages, of life. But the constant is that a woman is always female. Properly nourishing her feminine organs can often help her better maintain (and improve) her health.

Feminine Advantage™ is a 100% Food supplement that is intended to supply nutrients, glandulars, and herbs needed to maintain and support optimal female health.

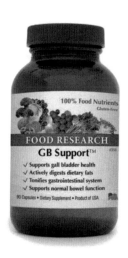

GB Support™

#356
90 Capsules

√ Supports gall bladder health

√ Actively digests dietary fats

√ Tonifies gastrointestinal system

√ Supports normal bowel function

Supplement Facts
Serving Size 1 Capsule   Servings per Container 90

Amount per Serving		% Daily Value▼	
Bovine Liver Cytotrophin		50 mg	*
Bovine Ox Bile		100 mg	*
Collinsonia Root	Collinsonia Canadensis	200 mg	*
Organic Carrot Root	Daucus Carota	50 mg	*
Wildcrafted Beet Root	Beta Vulgaris	30 mg	*

* Recommended Daily Intake has not been established

Other ingredients: Vegetarian (HPMC) Capsule.

Suggested use: Serving size or as recommended by your health care professional. Adjust usage according to nutritional lifestyle requirements.

GB Support™ is a 100% Food supplement that is intended to supply nutrients, glandulars, and herbs needed to maintain and support optimal gall bladder and digestive health.

GB Support™ provides bile that will support the healthy metabolism and absorption of dietary fat when the gall bladder has been surgically removed. Collinsonia root has long been used as a tonic herb to support the digestive system.

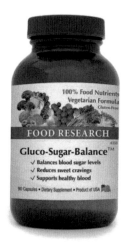

Gluco-Sugar-Balance™

#358
90 Capsules

√ Balances blood sugar levels

√ Reduces sweet cravings

√ Supports healthy blood

Supplement Facts
Serving Size 1 Capsule   Servings per Container 90

Amount per Serving			% Daily Value▼	
Chromium GTF	(in 50 mg food)	100 mcg	330%	
Vanadium	(in 50 mg food)	50 mcg		*
Food Extracted Berberine HCL	(Plant Source)	70 mg		*
Food Extracted Bitter Melon	Momordica Charantia	25 mg		*
Food Extracted N-Acetyl-L-Cysteine	(Plant Source)	10 mg		*
Gymnema Sylvestre Leaf	Gymnema Sylvestre	75 mg		*
Organic Cinnamon Bark	Cinnamon Cassia	50 mg		*
Organic Fenugreek Seed	Trigonella Foenum-Graecum	35 mg		*

* Recommended Daily Intake has not been established

Other ingredients: Enzymatically Processed *Saccharomyces Cerevisiae*, Vegetarian (HPMC) Capsule.

Suggested use: Serving size or as recommended by your health care professional. Adjust usage according to nutritional lifestyle requirements.

 Halal   Pareve

Gluco-Sugar-Balance™ is a 100% vegan Food intended to help support a healthy balance of glucose in the body. It contains minerals, such as chromium GTF and vanadium, as well as herbs to nutritionally support the body's blood sugar systems and naturally occurring potassium, polysaccharides, CoQ10, glutathione, lipoic acid, trace minerals, enzymes, peptides, RNA/DNA, carbohydrates, lipids, proteins *(including all ten essential amino acids)*, protein chaperones, and the antioxidant superoxide dismutase as found in enzymatically processed *Saccharomyces cerevisiae* and the other listed foods.

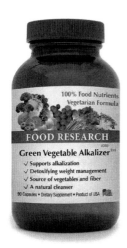

Green Vegetable Alkalizer™

#360
90 Capsules

√ Supports alkalization

√ Detoxifying weight management

√ Source of vegetables and fiber

√ A natural cleanser

Supplement Facts
Serving Size 1 Capsule Servings per Container 90

Amount per Serving		% Daily Value ▼	
Acid-Stabilized Enzymes		100 mg	*
Amylase, Cellulase, Invertase, Lactase, Lipase, Maltase, Protease I & II			
Organic Alfalfa Herb	Medicago Sativa	100 mg	*
Organic Barley Grass	Hordeum Vulgare L.	100 mg	*
Organic Celery Seed	Apium Graveolens	50 mg	*
Organic Parsley Leaf	Petroselinum Crispum	50 mg	*
Organic Wheatgrass	Elymus Trachycaulus	100 mg	*
Spinach Leaf	Spinacia Oleracea	25 mg	*
Wildcrafted Spirulina	Arthrospira Platensis	50 mg	*
Wildcrafted Watercress	Nasturtium Officinale	25 mg	*

* Recommended Daily Intake has not been established

Other ingredients: Silica, Vegetarian Capsule.

Suggested use: Serving size or as recommended by your health care professional. Adjust usage according to nutritional lifestyle requirements.

Green Vegetable Alkalizer™ is a 100% vegan Food supplement that is intended to supply 100% Food green alkalizing plants. Green vegetables are considered to be a natural cleanser for the digestive system and naturally contain nutrients that protect against free radicals.

Green Vegetable Alkalizer™ is a high quality, enzyme-containing mixture of green vegetables and concentrates.

 Vegetarian Formula

 Halal   Ⓟ Pareve

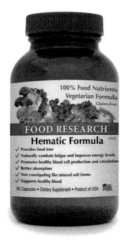

Hematic Formula™

#403
90 Capsules

√ Provides food iron

√ Naturally combats fatigue and improves energy levels

√ Promotes healthy blood cell production and circulation

√ Better absorption

√ Not constipating like mineral salt forms

√ Supports healthy blood

Supplement Facts
Serving Size 1 Capsule Servings per Container 90

Amount per Serving			% Daily Value ▼	
Vitamin C	(in 60 mg food)	15 mg	16%	
Vitamin B-6	(in 8 mg food)	1.6 mg	94%	
Folate (Vitamin B-9)	(in 40 mg food)	400 mcg DFE	100%	
Vitamin B-12 – Methylated	(in 3.6 mg food)	18 mcg	750%	
Iron	(in 360 mg food)	18 mg	100%	
Citrus Bioflavonoids	(Pesticide/Herbicide free)	60 mg	*	
Wildcrafted Beet Root	(Beta Vulgaris)	28 mg	*	

* Recommended Daily Intake has not been established

Other ingredients: Enzymatically Processed *Saccharomyces Cerevisiae*, Vegetarian (HPMC) Capsule.

Suggested use: Serving size or as recommended by your health care professional. Adjust usage according to nutritional lifestyle requirements.

Hematic Formula™ is a 100% vegan Food supplement that is intended to supply nutrients needed to maintain and support optimal blood health. Iron is an important nutrient essential for the synthesis of hemoglobin and contains part of the enzymes needed for cell respiration. **Hematic Formula™** is not constipating like iron-salt supplements can be.

 Vegetarian Formula   GLUTEN FREE

 Halal   Ⓟ Pareve

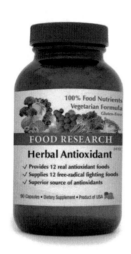

Herbal Antioxidant™

#410
90 Capsules

√ Provides 12 real antioxidant foods

√ Supplies 12 free-radical fighting foods

√ Superior source of antioxidants

Herbal Antioxidants™ is a 100% vegan Food supplement that is intended to supply real antioxidant nutrients needed to maintain and support optimal health and protection from free radicals.

Each of the antioxidant nutrients are 100% whole food and synergistically protect against a wide range of free radicals. Antioxidants are believed to help address the effects of aging, support healthy brain tissue, maintain capillary integrity, restore collagen strength, supports healthy skin, and maintain a healthy cardiovascular system.

Supplement Facts

Serving Size 1 Capsule   Servings per Container 90

Amount per Serving				% Daily Value ▼
Vitamin A (Betacarotene)	(in	40 mg food)	600 rae	66%
Vitamin C	(in	160 mg food)	40 mg	44%
Vitamin E	(in	50 mg food)	12 mg	83%
Zinc	(in	60 mg food)	3 mg	27%
Selenium	(in	17 mg food)	17 mcg	30%
Citrus Bioflavonoids	(Pesticide/Herbicide Free)		140 mg	*
Milk Thistle Seed	Silybum Marianum		13 mg	*
Acerola Cherry	Malpighia Glabra		20 mg	*
Wildcrafted Eleuthero Root	Eluetherococcus Senticosus		10 mg	*
Wildcrafted Ginger Root (Powder)	Zingiber Officinale		10 mg	*
Wildcrafted Ginkgo Leaf	Ginkgo Biloba		10 mg	*
Wildcrafted Rosemary Leaf	Rosemarinus Officinales		10 mg	*
Wildcrafted Schisandra Fruit	Schisandra Chinesis		10 mg	*
Wildcrafted Turmeric Root	Curcuma Domestica		10 mg	*

* Recommended Daily Intake has not been established

Other ingredients: Enzymatically Processed *Saccharomyces Cerevisiae*, Vegetarian (HPMC) Capsule.

Suggested use: Serving size or as recommended by your health care professional. Adjust usage according to nutritional lifestyle requirements.

 Vegetarian Formula

 Halal   Pareve

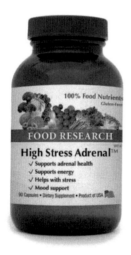

High Stress Adrenal™

#414
90 Capsules

√ Supports adrenal health

√ Supports energy

√ Helps with stress

√ Mood support

The adrenal glands play a role in energy, stress, mood, immune support, and pain management. **High Stress Adrenal™** is a 100% Food supplement that is intended to supply nutrients, glandulars, and herbs needed to maintain and support optimal adrenal health.

High Stress Adrenal™ contains many of the substances produced by, or naturally in, those glands including peptides, hormone precursors, and enzymes. Additionally, it includes l-tyrosine, food B vitamins, food vitamin C, and herbs to support healthy adrenal function.

Supplement Facts

Serving Size 3 Capsules   Servings per Container 30

Amount per Serving				% Daily Value ▼
Vitamin C	(in	272 mg food)	68 mg	75%
Thiamin (Vitamin B-1)	(in	17 mg food)	4 mg	340%
Riboflavin (Vitamin B-2)	(in	40 mg food)	4 mg	307%
Niacinamide (Vitamin B-3)	(in	80 mg food)	20 mg NE	125%
Vitamin B-6	(in	30 mg food)	6 mg	352%
Folate (Vitamin B-9)	(in	20 mg food)	200 mcg DFE	50%
Vitamin B-12 - Methylated	(in	2.4 mg food)	12 mcg	500%
Pantothenate (Vitamin B-5)	(in	120 mg food)	30 mg	600%
Choline	(in	12 mg food)	3 mg	*
Zinc	(in	60 mg food)	3 mg	27%
Inositol	(in	12 mg food)	3 mg	*
Acerola Cherry	Malpighia Glabra		40 mg	**
Bovine Adrenal Cytotrophin			150 mg	**
Bovine Hypothalamus Cytotrophin			15 mg	**
Citrus Bioflavonoids	(Pesticide/Herbicide Free)		232 mg	**
Food Extracted L-Tyrosine			354 mg	**
Organic Brown Rice	Oryza Sativa		6 mg	**
Wildcrafted Eleuthro Root	Eleutherococcus Senticosus		24 mg	**
Wildcrafted Kelp Thallus	Ascophyllum Nodosum		9 mg	**

* Contains less than 2% of the RDI   ** Recommended Daily Intake has not been established

Other ingredients: Enzymatically Processed *Saccharomyces Cerevisiae*, Vegetarian (HPMC) Capsule.

Suggested use: Serving size or as recommended by your health care professional. Adjust usage according to nutritional lifestyle requirements.

Hypothalamus EMG™

#440
90 Capsules

√ Supports healthy hypothalamus function

√ Calming

√ Supports the master endocrine gland

√ Promotes positive mood

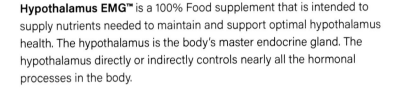

Supplement Facts
Serving Size 1 Capsule   Servings per Container 90

Amount per Serving		% Daily Value ▼
Bovine Hypothalamus Cytotrophin		30 mg	•
Collinsonia Root Powder	Collinsonia Canadensis	30 mg	•
Bovine Chymotrypsin		0.016 mg	•
Bovine Trypsin		0.007 mg	•

* Recommended Daily Intake has not been established

Other ingredients: Organic Brown Rice, Vegetarian (HPMC) Capsule.

Suggested use: Serving size or as recommended by your health care professional. Adjust usage according to nutritional lifestyle requirements.

Hypothalamus EMG™ is a 100% Food supplement that is intended to supply nutrients needed to maintain and support optimal hypothalamus health. The hypothalamus is the body's master endocrine gland. The hypothalamus directly or indirectly controls nearly all the hormonal processes in the body.

Hypothalamus EMG™ contains an Enzomorphogen extract which is uniquely derived in order to support cellular health.

Inflam-Enzymes™

#450
90 Tablets

√ Muscle detoxification

√ Improves flexibility

√ Relieves discomfort

√ Joint detoxification

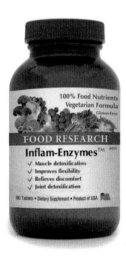

Supplement Facts
Serving Size 1 Tablet   Servings per Container 90

Amount per Serving			% Daily Value ▼
Vitamin C	(in | 15 mg food)	3.75 mg	4%
Calcium	(in | 40 mg food)	2 mg	*
Magnesium	(in | 40 mg food)	2 mg	*
Manganese	(in | 100 mg food)	5 mg	217%
Acerola Cherry	Malpighia Glabra	15 mg	**
Food Extracted Bromelain (from Pineapple)	Ananas Comosus	100 mg	**
Food Extracted Papain (from Papaya)	Carica Papaya	100 mg	**
Serrapeptase (Enzyme)	Serratia Peptidase	10 mg	**
Wildcrafted Astragalus Root	Astragalus Membranaceus	100 mg	**

* Contains less than 2% of the RDI
** Recommended Daily Intake has not been established

Other ingredients: Enzymatically Processed *Saccharomyces Cerevisiae,* Vegetable Oil Extract.

Suggested use: Serving size or as recommended by your health care professional. Adjust usage according to nutritional lifestyle requirements.

 Vegetarian Formula

 Halal   Pareve

Many people have inflammation in the discs of their back, their muscles, and various joints in the body. In addition to pain, inflammation can result in damage to soft tissues.

Inflam-Enzymes™ is a 100% Food supplement that is intended to supply nutrients, enzymes, glandulars, and herbs needed to maintain and support optimal ligament and tendon health. This product was designed for chiropractors and other doctors interested in relieving back and soft tissue discomfort.

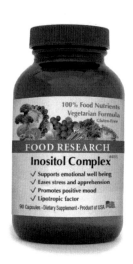

Inositol Complex™

#455
90 Capsules

√ Supports emotional well-being

√ Eases stress and apprehension

√ Promotes positive mood

√ Lipotropic factor

Supplement Facts
Serving Size 1 Capsule   Servings per Container 90

Amount per Serving		% Daily Value ▼
Inositol	(in 440 mg food)	110 mg	
Okra (Fruit)	Abelmoschus Esculentus	30 mg	

* Recommended Daily Intake has not been established

Other ingredients: Enzymatically processed *Saccharomyces Cerevisiae*, Organic Brown Rice, Vegetarian (HPMC) Capsule.

Suggested use: Serving size or as recommended by your health care professional. Adjust usage according to nutritional lifestyle requirements.

Inositol Complex™ is a 100% vegetarian Food supplement that is intended to supply real food Inositol. Inositol supports emotional well-being, eases stress, and promotes a positive mood. Inositol has been used as nutritional support for people with brain, kidney, bone marrow, skin, hair, mood, muscular control, and blood cholesterol concerns.

Inositol was once called vitamin B-8. It is a lipotropic factor, a chelater, and seems to have positive effects on the immune system. It also shares many of Choline's functions.

 Vegetarian Formula

 Halal   Pareve

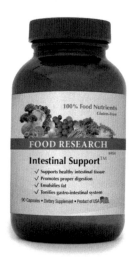

Intestinal Support™

#454
90 Capsules

√ Supports healthy intestinal tissue

√ Promotes proper digestion

√ Emulsifies fat

√ Tonifies gastro-intestinal system

Supplement Facts
Serving Size 1 Capsule   Servings per Container 90

Amount per Serving		% Daily Value ▼
Bovine Intestinal Cytotrophin		45 mg	
Bovine Liver Cytotrophin		50 mg	
Bovine Lymph Cytotrophin		100 mg	
Bovine Ox Bile		20 mg	
Bovine Pancreas Cytotrophin		75 mg	
Wildcrafted Cinnamon Bark	Cinnamon Cassia	20 mg	
Wildcrafted Collinsonia Root	Collinsonia Canadensis	90 mg	

* Recommended Daily Intake has not been established

Other ingredients: Vegetarian (HPMC) Capsule.

Suggested use: Serving size or as recommended by your health care professional. Adjust usage according to nutritional lifestyle requirements.

Intestinal Support™ is a 100% Food supplement contains herbs and other glandular to support intestinal and digestive health.

Intestines are involved in the digestion and absorption of nutrients as well as the excretion of waste. When they are not functioning well there can be digestive problems. If they are weak, hernias and/or colorectal issues sometimes develop. Bovine intestinal tissue provides peptides and enzymes to nutritionally support the intestines.

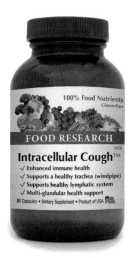

Intracellular Cough™

#458
90 Capsules

√ Enhanced immune health

√ Supports a healthy trachea (windpipe)

√ Supports healthy lymphatic system

√ Multi-glandular health support

Supplement Facts
Serving Size 1 Capsule   Servings per Container 90

Amount per Serving		% Daily Value ▼
Vitamin C	(in 50 mg food)	12.5 mg 13%
Bovine Heart Cytotrophin		65 mg
Bovine Hypothalamus Cytotrophin		2 mg
Bovine Liver Cytotrophin		20 mg
Bovine Lymph Cytotrophin		20 mg
Bovine Parathyroid Cytotrophin		1 mg
Bovine Pineal Cytotrophin		1 mg
Bovine Pituitary Cytotrophin		0.3 mg
Bovine Spleen Cytotrophin		12 mg
Bovine Thymus Cytotrophin		35 mg
Bovine Thyroid Cytotrophin		7 mg
Bovine Trachea Cytotrophin		4 mg
Acerola Cherry	Malpighia Glabra	50 mg
Bromelain (Pineapple Source)	Ananas Comosus	100 mg
Elderberry Flower	Sambucus Nigra	28 mg
Organic Brown Rice	Oryza Sativa	70 mg
Organic Carrot Root	Daucus Carota	30 mg
Sunflower Lecithin	Helianthus Annuus	30 mg
Wildcrafted Icelandic Moss	Cetraria Islandica	10 mg
Wildcrafted Juniper Berries	Juniperus Communis	9 mg
Wildcrafted Passion Flower	Passiflora Incarnata	7 mg
Wildcrafted Uva Ursi	Arctostaphylos Uva-Ursi	8 mg

* Recommended Daily Intake has not been established

Other ingredients: Vegetarian (HPMC) Capsule.

Suggested use: Serving size or as recommended by your health care professional. Adjust usage according to nutritional lifestyle requirements.

Intracellular Cough™ is a 100% Food supplement that is intended to supply nutrients, glandulars, and herbs needed to maintain and support optimal immune system health.

Intracellular Cough™ is a pluriglandular formula that supports many of the body's systems. This multi-glandular formula also includes immune system supporting herbs.

Kidney Support™

#459
90 Capsules

√ Supports healthy kidneys

√ Supports proper fluid balance

√ Supports a healthy urinary system

Supplement Facts
Serving Size 1 Capsule   Servings per Container 90

Amount per Serving		% Daily Value ▼
Vitamin C	(in 120 mg food)	30 mg 33%
Acerola Cherry	Malphighia glabra	120 mg
Bovine Kidney Cytotrophin		100 mg
Bovine Liver Cytotrophin		50 mg
Bovine Pancreas Cytotrophin		10 mg
Buckwheat Grain	Fagopyrum Esculentum	50 mg
Cat's Claw	Uncaria Tomentosa	30 mg
Corn Silk Extract 4:1	Zea Mays	20 mg
Dandelion Root	Taraxacum Officinale	20 mg
Garlic	Allium Sativum	10 mg
Organic Carrot Root	Daucus Carota	20 mg
Red Clover	Trifolium Pratense	30 mg
Wildcrafted Beet Root	Beta Vulgaris	40 mg

* Recommended Daily Intake has not been established

Other ingredients: Vegetarian (HPMC) Capsule.

Suggested use: Serving size or as recommended by your health care professional. Adjust usage according to nutritional lifestyle requirements.

Kidney Support™ is a 100% Food supplement that is intended to supply nutrients to support healthy kidney and urinary system function. The kidneys process proteins and liquids and are the primary organs involved in eliminating metabolic waste products from the blood.

Kidney Support™ is intended to support the healthy functioning of the kidneys.

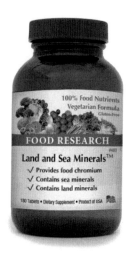

Land and Sea Minerals™

#460
180 Tablets

√ Provides food chromium

√ Contains sea minerals

√ Contains land minerals

Supplement Facts
Serving Size 1 Tablet   Servings per Container 180

Amount per Serving			% Daily Value ▼
Chromium GTF	(in 5 mg food)	10 mcg	33%
Wildcrafted Alfalfa Juice (Dried)	Medicago Sativa	335 mg	*
Wildcrafted Kelp Thallus	Ascophyllum Nodosum	200 mcg	*

* Recommended Daily Intake has not been established

Other ingredients: Enzymatically Processed *Saccharomyces Cerevisiae*, Vegetarian (HPMC) Capsule.

Suggested use: Serving size or as recommended by your health care professional. Adjust usage according to nutritional lifestyle requirements.

Land and Sea Minerals™ is a multi-mineral product containing potassium and a variety of alkaline ash minerals. Potassium is important for healthy function of bodily systems such as cardiovascular and parasympathetic nervous systems.

Many systems of the body not only require potassium but also trace minerals, which are naturally found in foods such as kelp and alfalfa.

 Vegetarian Formula   GLUTEN FREE

 Halal   Pareve

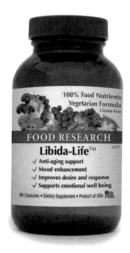

Libida-Life™

#477
90 Capsules

√ Anti-aging support

√ Mood enhancement

√ Improves desire and response

√ Supports emotional well-being

Supplement Facts
Serving Size 1 Capsule   Servings per Container 90

Amount per Serving			% Daily Value ▼
Zinc	(in 44 mg food)	2.2 mg	20%
Selenium	(in 14 mg food)	14 mcg	25%
Food Extracted L-Arginine (Plant Source)		50 mg	*
Food Extracted L-Ornithine (Plant Source)		10 mg	*
Milk Thistle Seed (Naturally Contains Silymarin)	Silybin Marianum	20 mg	*
Resveratrol (from Grape Skin)		50 mg	*
Wildcrafted Astragalus Root	Astragalus Membranaceus	68 mg	*
Wildcrafted Maca	Lepidum Meyenii	140 mg	*

* Recommended Daily Intake has not been established

Other ingredients: Enzymatically Processed *Saccharomyces Cerevisiae*, Vegetarian (HPMC) Capsule.

Suggested use: Serving size or as recommended by your health care professional. Adjust usage according to nutritional lifestyle requirements.

Libida-Life™ is a 100% Food supplement that is intended to have anti-aging properties and support a healthy sexual response system. It contains minerals, herbs, and the amino acid l-arginine.

Libida-Life™ contains naturally occurring potassium, polysaccharides, CoQ10, glutathione, lipoic acid, trace minerals, enzymes, peptides, RNA/DNA, carbohydrates, lipids, proteins (including all ten essential amino acids), protein chaperones, and the antioxidant superoxide dismutase as found in Saccharomyces cerevisiae.

 Vegetarian Formula   GLUTEN FREE

 Halal   Pareve

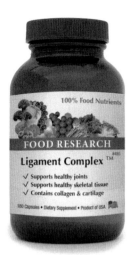

Ligament Complex™

#485
180 Capsules

√ Supports healthy joints
√ Supports healthy skeletal tissue
√ Contains collagen & cartilage

Supplement Facts				
Serving Size 1 Capsule Servings per Container 180				
Amount per Serving			**% Daily Value ▼**	
Vitamin A (Betacarotene)	(in	5 mg food)	75 rae	8%
Vitamin C	(in	6 mg food)	1.5 mg	*
Vitamin D	(in	.5 mg food)	500 i.u.	62%
Vitamin E	(in	5 mg food)	1.25 mg	8%
Vitamin B-12 – Methylated	(in	3.2 mg food)	1.60 mcg	66%
Calcium	(in	25 mg food)	1.25 mg	*
Manganese	(in	25 mg food)	1.25 mg	54%
Inositol	(in	1 mg food)	250 mcg	*
PABA (Para-aminobenzoic Acid)	(in	5 mg food)	2.88 mg	*
Acerola Cherry	*Malpighia Glabra*		6 mg	**
Bovine Adrenal Cytotrophin			30 mg	**
Bovine Bone Marrow			5 mg	**
Bovine Bone Meal			20 mg	**
Bovine Cartilage			10 mg	**
Bovine Collagen Peptides			35 mg	**
Bovine Heart Cytotrophin			20 mg	**
Bovine Kidney Cytotrophin			20 mg	**
Bovine Liver Cytotrophin			60 mg	**
Bovine Spleen Cytotrophin			39 mg	**
Natural Carbamide			10 mg	**
Organic Brown Rice	*Oryza Sativa*		20 mg	**
Organic Carrot Root	*Daucus Carota*		10 mg	**
Organic Flaxseeds	*Linum Usitatissimum*		20 mg	**
Organic Shiitake Mushroom	*Lentinula Edodes*		10 mg	**
Ribonucleic Acid			5 mg	**
Sunflower Lecithin	*Helianthus Annuus*		10 mg	**
Wheat Germ (Defatted)	*Triticum Aestivum*		10 mg	**
Wildcrafted Beet Root	*Beta Vulgaris*		10 mg	**
Wildcrafted Icelandic Moss	*Cetraria Islandica*		25 mg	**
Wildcrafted Wheatgrass	*Elymus Trachycaulus*		10 mg	**
* Contains less than 2% of the RDI				
** Recommended Daily Intake has not been established				

Other ingredients: Enzymatically Processed *Saccharomyces Cerevisiae*, Vegetarian (HPMC) Capsule.

Suggested use: Serving size or as recommended by your health care professional. Adjust usage according to nutritional lifestyle requirements.

Ligament Complex™ helps support healthy ligaments and encourages healthy long term tissue support for athletes. Ligaments are strong fibrous cords which are mainly made up of collagen fibers. Calcium supports healthy bones.

Many of the nutrients in Ligament Complex™ support healthy joints.

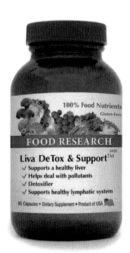

Liva-DeTox & Support™

#496
90 Capsules

√ Supports a healthy liver
√ Helps deal with pollutants
√ Detoxifier
√ Supports healthy lymphatic system

Supplement Facts			
Serving Size 1 Capsule Servings per Container 90			
Amount per Serving		**% Daily Value ▼**	
Bovine Liver Cytotrophin		170 mg	*
Bovine Spleen Cytotrophin		20 mg	*
Garlic Bulb	*Allium Sativa*	40 mg	*
Milk Thistle Seed (Naturally Contains Silymarin)	*Silybin Marianum*	100 mg	*
Wildcrafted Beet Root	*Beta Vulgaris*	20 mg	*
* Recommended Daily Intake has not been established			

Other ingredients: Vegetarian (HPMC) Capsule.

Suggested use: Serving size or as recommended by your health care professional. Adjust usage according to nutritional lifestyle requirements.

Liva-DeTox & Support™ is a 100% Food supplement that is intended to supply nutrients, glandulars, and herbs needed to maintain and support optimal liver health.

Liva-DeTox & Support™ naturally contains carbohydrates, lipids, and proteins (including all ten essential amino acids), and protein chaperones as found in the listed foods—all the nutrients shown above are contained in these foods.

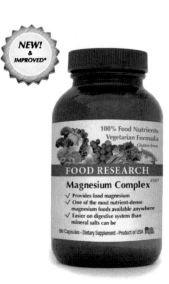

Magnesium Complex™

#567 – Small/90C
#568 – Large/270C

√ Provides food magnesium

√ One of the most nutrient-dense magnesium foods available anywhere

√ Easier on digestive system than mineral salts can be

Supplement Facts

Serving Size 3 Capsules   Servings per Container 30

Amount per Serving		% Daily Value ▼	
Magnesium	(in 1400 mg food)	168 mg	40%
Biogurt (Lactobacillus Bulgaricus)		1292 mg	*
Wildcrafted Spinach Leaf	(Spinacia Oleracea)	108 mg	*

* Recommended Daily Intake has not been established

Other ingredients: Organic Brown Rice, Vegetarian (HPMC) Capsule.

Suggested use: Serving size or as recommended by your health care professional. Adjust usage according to nutritional lifestyle requirements.

Now in Capsules • Easier to Swallow

29.2% *More Magnesium per bottle!*

 Vegetarian Formula

 GLUTEN FREE

 Halal

 Pareve

Magnesium Complex™ is a 100% vegan Food supplement that is intended to supply 100% Food magnesium.

Clinical deficiency of magnesium can results in "depressed tendon reflexes, muscle fasciculations, tremor, muscle spasm, personality changes, anorexia, nausea, and vomiting". Magnesium deficiency reportedly produces hypercholesterolemia, hypertriglyceridemia, and dyslipoproteinemia by increasing VLDL and low density lipoprotein, and decreasing high density lipoprotein cholesterol.

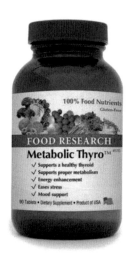

Metabolic Thyro™

#570

90 Tablets

√ Supports a healthy thyroid

√ Supports proper metabolism

√ Energy enhancement

√ Eases stress

√ Mood support

Supplement Facts

Serving Size 1 Tablet   Servings per Container 90

Amount per Serving		% Daily Value ▼	
Chromium GTF	(in 12.5 mg food)	25 mcg	83%
Bovine Adrenal Cytotrophin		10 mg	*
Bovine Liver Cytotrophin		30 mg	*
Bovine Pituitary Cytotrophin		1 mg	*
Bovine Thyroid Cytotrophin		50 mg	*
Food Extracted L-Tyrosine	(Vegan GMO-Free)	50 mg	*
Organic Alfalfa (Aerial Parts)	Medicago Sativa	13 mg	*
Organic Burdock Root	Arctium Lappa	50 mg	*
Organic Fenugreek Seed	Trigonella Foenum-Graecum	250 mcg	*
Organic Shiitake Mushroom	Lentinula Edodes	250 mcg	*
Scullcap (Root Extract)	Scutellaria Baicalensis	10 mg	*
Wildcrafted Broccoli	Brassica Oleracea	13 mg	*
Wildcrafted Kelp Thallus	Ascophyllum Nodosum	25 mg	*

* Recommended Daily Intake has not been established

Other ingredients: Plant Polysaccharides, Silica, Vegetable Oil Extract.

Suggested use: Serving size or as recommended by your health care professional. Adjust usage according to nutritional lifestyle requirements.

 GLUTEN FREE

Metabolic Thyro™ is a 100% Food supplement that is intended to supply nutrients, glandulars, and herbs needed to maintain and support optimal thyroid health. It comprises both natural-iodine containing kelp, plant source l-tyrosine, bovine glandulars, and herbs to support an optimally functioning thyroid.

Metabolic Thyro™ naturally contains carbohydrates (including all known essential monosaccharides), essential lipids, and proteins (including all ten essential amino acids) as found in specially grown, enzymatically processed Saccharomyces cerevisiae and the individually listed foods.

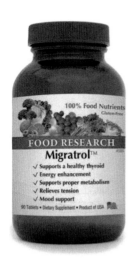

Migratrol™

#585
90 Tablets

√ Supports a healthy thyroid
√ Energy enhancement
√ Supports proper metabolism
√ Relieves tension
√ Mood support

Migratrol™ is a 100% Food supplement that is intended to supply nutrients, glandulars, and herbs needed to maintain and support optimal thyroid health. A mild product that often is used by older people and some with headaches.

Migratrol™ contains carbohydrates (including all known essential monosaccharides), essential lipids, and proteins (including all ten essential amino acids) as found in specially grown, enzymatically processed Saccharomyces cerevisiae and the individually listed foods. All glandulars are New Zealand source.

Supplement Facts
Serving Size 1 Tablet   Servings per Container 90

Amount per Serving			% Daily Value ▼	
Riboflavin (Vitamin B-2)	(in	17 mg food)	1.7 mg	100%
Niacinamide (Vitamin B-3)	(in	40 mg food)	10 mg NE	62%
Magnesium	(in	280 mg food)	14 mg	3%
Chromium GTF	(in	5 mg food)	10 mcg	3%
Bovine Adrenal (Suprarenal) Cytotrophin			15 mg	*
Bovine Liver Cytotrophin			10 mg	*
Bovine Pituitary Cytotrophin			200 mcg	*
Bovine Thyroid Cytotrophin			25 mg	*
Dong Quai Root		Angelica Sinensis	50 mg	*
Organic Flaxseeds		Linum Usitatissimum	25 mg	*
Wildcrafted Feverfew Leaf		Tanacetum Parthenium	25 mg	*

* Recommended Daily Intake has not been established

Other ingredients: Croscarmellose Sodium *(Digestive Aid)*, Enzymatically processed *Saccharomyces Cerevisiae*, Silica, Vegetable Oil Extract.

Suggested use: Serving size or as recommended by your health care professional. Adjust usage according to nutritional lifestyle requirements.

Not Recommended During Pregnancy.

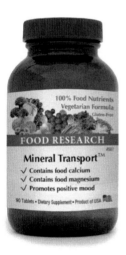

Mineral Transport™

#587
90 Tablets

√ Contains food calcium
√ Contains food magnesium
√ Promotes positive mood

Mineral Transport™ is a formula that contains nutrients that can work together as a mild calmative. Calcium and magnesium can help establish a more balanced central nervous system. Calcium and magnesium also are involved in supporting healthy muscle function.

Supplement Facts
Serving Size 1 Tablet   Servings per Container 90

Amount per Serving			% Daily Value ▼	
Calcium	(in	250 mg food)	30 mg	*
Magnesium	(in	100 mg food)	12 mg	*
Alfalfa Leaf		Medicago Sativa	25 mg	**
Biogurt (Lactobacillus Bulgaricus)			350 mg	**
Parsley Leaf		Petroselinum Crispum	20 mg	**
Wildcrafted Kelp Thallus		Ascophyllum Nodosum	50 mcg	**

* Contains less than 2% of the RDI
** Recommended Daily Intake has not been established

Other ingredients: Croscarmellose Sodium *(Digestive Aid)*, Silica, Vegetable Oil Extract. Contains No Magnesium Stearate.

Suggested use: Serving size or as recommended by your health care professional. Adjust usage according to nutritional lifestyle requirements.

 Vegetarian Formula

 Halal
 Pareve

P
R
O
D
U
C
T
S

L
A
B
E
L

I
N
F
O
R
M
A
T
I
O
N

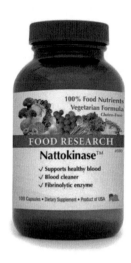

Nattokinase™

#590
100 Capsules

√ Supports healthy blood
√ Blood cleaner
√ Fibrinolytic enzyme

Supplement Facts

Serving Size 2 Capsules   Servings per Container 50

Amount per Serving	% Daily Value▼
Nattokinase *(Fermented Soy Extract 1,440 Fibrin Units)*	72 mg *

* Recommended Daily Intake has not been established

Other ingredients: Vegetarian (HPMC) Capsule, Wildcrafted Beet Root.

Suggested use: Serving size or as recommended by your health care professional. Adjust usage according to nutritional lifestyle requirements.

Nattokinase™ is a 100% vegan Food supplement that is intended to supply nutrients needed to provide high quality vegan nattokinase. Nattokinase is considered to be a fibrinolytic enzyme. It is capable of directly activating pro-urokinase (endogenous) and decomposing fibrin. Nattokinase assists in the body's fibrinolytic activity, supports cadiovascular health, and supports circulation.

Natto is a vegetable cheese-like food which is extremely popular in Japan. It has been around at least 1000 years.

 Vegetarian Formula GLUTEN FREE

 Halal Pareve

Nerve Chex B™

#597
90 Capsules

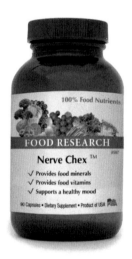

√ Provides food minerals
√ Provides food vitamins
√ Supports a healthy mood

Supplement Facts

Serving Size 1 Capsule   Servings per Container 90

Amount per Serving			% Daily Value▼	
Vitamin C	(in	12 mg food)	3 mg	3%
Vitamin B-1 (Thiamine)	(in	4 mg food)	1 mg	83%
Vitamin G (Riboflavin B-2)	(in	13 mg food)	1.3 mg	100%
Vitamin B-3 (Niacinamide)	(in	100 mg food)	25 mg NE	156%
Vitamin B-6	(in	25 mg food)	5 mg	294%
Vitamin B-12 – Methylated	(in	.3 mg food)	1.5 mcg	62%
Choline	(in	4 mg food)	1 mg	•
Calcium	(in	20 mg food)	1 mg	•
Magnesium	(in	50 mg food)	2.5 mg	•
Manganese	(in	10 mg food)	.5 mg	25%
Acerola Cherry	*Malpighia Glabra*		12 mg	**
Betaine HCL			14 mg	**
Bovine Brain Cytotrophin			5 mg	**
Bovine Hypothalamus Cytotrophin			20 mg	**
Bovine Liver Cytotrophin			30 mg	**
Bovine Orchic Cytotrophin			80 mg	**
Bovine Spleen Cytotrophin			30 mg	**
Kelp Thallus	*Ascophyllum Nodosum*		200 mcg	**
PABA (Para-aminobenzoic Acid)	(in	10 mg food)	5.04 mg	**
Wheat Germ (Defatted)	*Triticum Aestivum*		10 mg	**

* Contains less than 2% of the RDI
** Recommended Daily Intake has not been established

Other ingredients: Enzymatically processed *Saccharomyces Cerevisiae*, Vegetarian (HPMC) Capsule.

Suggested use: Serving size or as recommended by your health care professional. Adjust usage according to nutritional lifestyle requirements.

Nerve Chex B™ is a supplement complex intended to function synergistically as a moderate calmative. Some of its ingredients like vitamin C from acerola cherries, support healthy adrenal gland function.

Nerve Chex B™ has been formulated with a combination of vitamins, minerals, herbs and glandulars to support a healthy mood.

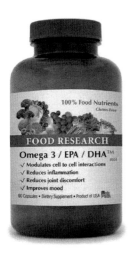

Omega 3 / EPA / DHA™

#604
90 Gelcaps

√ Modulates cell to cell interactions

√ Reduces inflammation

√ Reduces joint discomfort

√ Improves mood

Supplement Facts
Serving Size 1 Gelcap   Servings per Container 90

Amount per Serving			% Daily Value ▼
Vitamin E	(in 1000 mg food)	3.3 mg	22%
Docosahexaenoic Acid - DHA	(in 1000 mg Food)	120 mg	*
Eicosapentaenoic Acid – EPA	(in 1000 mg Food)	180 mg	*
Wild Herring Fish Oil		1000 mg	*

* Recommended Daily Intake has not been established

Other ingredients: Bovine Gelatin Capsule, Glycerin, Purified Water.

Suggested use: Serving size or as recommended by your health care professional. Adjust usage according to nutritional lifestyle requirements.

Omega 3/EPA/DHA™ is a 100% Whole Food supplement that is intended to supply nutrients needed to provide high quality herring source essential fatty acids like omega 3 as well as EPA, DHA, and support factors. In addition to their structural roles, essential fatty acids modulate cell to cell interactions.

There are many types of fish oil products on the market. The good ones have high contents of EPA and DHA but the best ones also contain oil from wild herring (or similar fish) that has been molecularly distilled to eliminate heavy metal concerns.

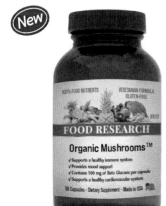

Organic Mushrooms™

#610
90 Capsules

√ Supports a healthy immune system

√ Provides mood support

√ Contains 80 mg of beta glucans per capsule

√ Supports a healthy cardiovascular system

Supplement Facts
Serving Size 1 Capsule   Servings per Container 90

Amount per Serving			% Daily Value ▼
Organic Cordyceps	Cordyceps Militaris	100 mg	*
Organic Lion's Mane	Hericium Erinaceus	100 mg	*
Organic Chaga	Inonotus Obliquus	50 mg	*
Organic Reishi	Ganoderma Lucidum	50 mg	*
Organic Shiitake	Lentinula Edodes	50 mg	*
Organic Turkey Tail (8:1 concetrate)	Trametes Versicolor	50 mg	*

* Recommended Daily Intake has not been established

Other ingredients: Vegetarian (HPMC) Capsule.

Suggested use: Serving size or as recommended by your health care professional. Adjust usage according to nutritional lifestyle requirements.

Organic Mushrooms supplies a healthy immune supporting blend of Organic Chaga (*Inonotus obliquus*), Organic Cordyceps *Cordyceps militaris*, Organic Lion's Mane *Hericium erinaceus*, Organic Reishi *Ganoderma lucidum*, Organic Shiitake *Lentinula edodes*, and Organic Turkey Tail *Trametes versicolor* which naturally provides beta glucans.

 Vegetarian Formula

 Halal Pareve

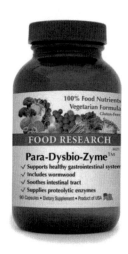

Para-Dysbio-Zyme™

#621
90 Capsules

√ Supports healthy gastrointestinal system

√ Includes wormwood

√ Soothes intestinal tract

√ Supplies proteolytic enzymes

Supplement Facts
Serving Size 2 Capsules   Servings per Container 45

Amount per Serving		% Daily Value ▼
Almond Meal (Raw)	Prunus Dulcis	150 mg *
Bromelain	Ananas Comosus	5 mg *
Burdock Root	Articium Lappa	30 mg *
Food Extracted Cellulase		5 mg *
Food Extracted Lipase		5 mg *
Garlic	Allium Sativa	30 mg *
Grapefruit Seed Extract	Citrus x Paradisi	20 mg *
Organic Carrot Root	Daucus Carota	20 mg *
Organic Cloves	Syzgium Aromaticum	10 mg *
Wildcrafted Astragalus Root	Astragalus Membranaceus	25 mg *
Wildcrafted Black Walnut (Inner Hull)	Juglans Nigra	50 mg *
Wildcrafted Fig	Ficum Carcica	50 mg *
Wildcrafted Wormwood Leaf (Powder)	Artemisia Absinthium	100 mg *

* Recommended Daily Intake has not been established

Other ingredients: Vegetarian (HPMC) Capsule.

Suggested use: Serving size or as recommended by your health care professional. Adjust usage according to nutritional lifestyle requirements.

Not Recommended During Pregnancy.

 Halal Pareve

Para-Dysbio-Zyme™ is a 100% Food vegan supplement that is intended to supply enzymes and herbs needed to maintain and support optimal digestive health. It provides herbs and various proteolytic enzymes to support the healthy functioning of the gastrointestinal system.

Unlike many so-called "natural" formulas, **Para-Dysbio-Zyme™** is only comprised of foods. It does not contain any synthetic USP nutrients or isolated mineral salts, but only contains foods, food complexes, and food concentrates.

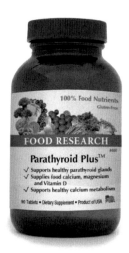

Parathyroid Plus™

#618
90 Tablets

√ Supports healthy parathyroid glands

√ Supplies food calcium and magnesium

√ Supplies food Vitamin D

√ Supports healthy calcium metabolism

Supplement Facts
Serving Size 1 Tablet   Servings per Container 90

Amount per Serving			% Daily Value ▼	
Vitamin D	(in	.5 mg food)	500 i.u.	62%
Calcium	(in	433 mg food)	52 mg	*
Magnesium	(in	60 mg food)	8 mg	*
Biogurt (Lactobacillus Bulgaricus)			493.5 mg	**
Bovine Parathyroid			2 mg	**

* Contains less than 2% of the RDI
** Recommended Daily Intake has not been established

Other ingredients: Croscarmellose Sodium (Digestive Aid), Enzymatically processed Saccharomyces Cerevisiae, Vegetable Oil Extract, Silica. Contains No Magnesium Stearate.

Suggested use: Serving size or as recommended by your health care professional. Adjust usage according to nutritional lifestyle requirements.

Parathyroid Plus™ is a parathyroid support product. The human body has four small parathyroid glands which are involved in the regulation of calcium metabolism.

Humans do not have proper calcium metabolism without properly functioning parathyroid glands. Calcium and magnesium help support healthy bones, nails, and joints.

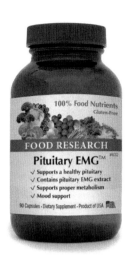

Pituitary EMG™

#632
90 Capsules

√ Supports a healthy pituitary

√ Contains pituitary EMG extract

√ Supports proper metabolism

√ Mood support

Supplement Facts
Serving Size 1 Capsule   Servings per Container 90

Amount per Serving		% Daily Value▼	
Bovine Pituitary Cytotrophin		30 mg	*
Collinsonia Root Powder	*Collinsonia Canadensis*	30 mg	*
Bovine Chymotrypsin		0.016 mg	*
Bovine Trypsin		0.007 mg	*
* Recommended Daily Intake has not been established			

Other ingredients: Organic Brown Rice, Vegetarian (HPMC) Capsule.

Suggested use: Serving size or as recommended by your health care professional. Adjust usage according to nutritional lifestyle requirements.

Pituitary EMG™ is a 100% Food supplement that is intended to supply nutrients needed to maintain and support optimal pituitary health. The pituitary is a major endocrine gland and is responsible for numerous hormones, including thyroid and gender related ones.

Pituitary EMG™ contains an Enzomorphogen extract which are uniquely derived in order to support cellular health.

All FOOD RESEARCH Products are 100% Food Nutrients!

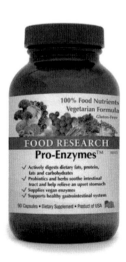

Pro-Enzymes™

#645
90 Capsules

√ Actively digest dietary fats, protein and carbohydrates

√ Probiotics and herbs soothe intestinal tract and help relieve an upset stomach

√ Supplies vegan enzymes

√ Supports healthy gastrointestinal system

Supplement Facts
Serving Size 1 Capsule   Servings per Container 90

Amount per Serving		% Daily Value▼	
Amylase (Enzyme)		7,000 DU	*
Cellulase (Enzyme)		100 CU	*
Invertase (Enzyme)		0.1 IAU	*
Lactase (Enzyme)		400 LacU	*
Lipase (Enzyme)		80 LU	*
Protease (Enzyme)		15,000 HUT	*
Gentian Root	*Gentiana Luten*	75 mg	*
Lactobacillus Acidophilus (Probiotic)		2,000,000 Units	*
Organic Ginger	*Zingiber Officinale*	30 mg	*
Pumpkin Seed	*Cucurbita Maxima*	45 mg	*
Wildcrafted Beet Root	*Beta Vulgaris*	240 mg	*
* Recommended Daily Intake has not been established			

Other ingredients: Silica, Vegetarian (HPMC) Capsule.

Suggested use: Serving size or as recommended by your health care professional. Adjust usage according to nutritional lifestyle requirements.

Pro-Enzymes™ is a 100% Food vegan supplement that is intended to supply plant source enzymes, probiotics, and herbs needed to maintain optimal and support digestive health. This is a true vegan digestive and probiotic support product.

Pro-Enzymes™ provides amylase for digesting starches, beet root and other herbs for fiber and digestive support.

 Vegetarian Formula

 Halal
 Pareve

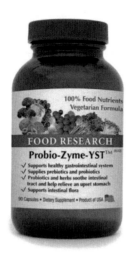

Probio-Zyme-YST™

#648
90 Capsules

√ Supports healthy gastrointestinal system

√ Supplies prebiotics and probiotics

√ Probiotics and herbs soothe intestinal tract and help relieve an upset stomach

√ Supports intestinal flora

Supplement Facts

Serving Size 1 Capsule   Servings per Container 90

Amount per Serving		% Daily Value ▼	
Zinc (in 30 mg food)		1.5 mg	13%
Lactobacillus Acidophilus		2,000,000 u	*
Cellulase (Enzyme)		200 cu	*
Cabbage Leaf	*Brassica Oleracea*	25 mg	*
Coconut Oil (Naturally containing Caprylic Acid)		70 mg	*
Citrus Aurantium Fruit		15 mg	*
Garlic	*Allium Sativum*	15 mg	*
Olive Leaf Extract	*Olea Europaea*	10 mg	*
Psyllium Husk	*Plantago Ovata*	10 mg	*
Sweet Violet Leaf	*Viola Odorata*	10 mg	*
Wheat Germ (Defatted)	*Triticum Aestivum*	70 mg	*
Wildcrafted Artichoke Leaf	*Cynara Scolomus*	10 mg	*
Wildcrafted Beet Root	*Beta Vulgaris*	20 mg	*
Wildcrafted Cinnamon Bark	*Cinnamomum Verum*	15 mg	*
Wildcrafted Cloves	*Syzygium Aromaticum*	8 mg	*
Wildcrafted Icelandic Moss	*Cetraria Islandica*	20 mg	*
Wildcrafted Oregano Leaf	*Origanum Vulgare*	26 mg	*

* Recommended Daily Intake has not been established

Other ingredients: Enzymatically processed *Saccharomyces Cerevisiae,* Silica, Vegetarian (HPMC) Capsule.

Suggested use: Serving size or as recommended by your health care professional. Adjust usage according to nutritional lifestyle requirements.

Probio-Zyme-YST™ is a 100% Food vegan supplement that is intended to supply enzymes, prebiotics, probiotics, and herbs needed to maintain and support optimal digestive health. It contains nutrients that aid in the maintenance, as well as establishment, of normal intestinal flora and proper pH.

Probio-Zyme-YST™ contains a variety of prebiotic, probiotic, and anti-fungal herbal ingredients. Products like it have long been used as intestinal detoxificants. Combining pre- and pro-biotics seems to enhance effectiveness.

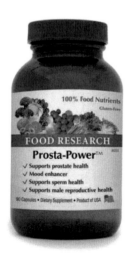

Prosta-Power™

#655
90 Capsules

√ Supports prostate health

√ Mood enhancer

√ Supports sperm health

√ Supports male reproductive health

Supplement Facts

Serving Size 1 Capsule   Servings per Container 90

Amount per Serving			% Daily Value ▼	
Vitamin E	(in	8 mg food)	1.34 mg	9%
Zinc	(in	8 mg food)	.40 mg	3%
Selenium	(in	18 mg food)	1 mcg	3%
African Pygeum	*Pygeum Africanum*		20 mg	*
Bovine Orchic Cytotrophin			80 mg	*
Bovine Prostate Cytotrophin			80 mg	*
Damiana Leaf	*Turnera Diffusa*		50 mg	*
Flaxseed	*Linum Usitatissimum*		20 mg	*
Korean Red Ginseng	*Panax Ginseng*		50 mg	*
Maca	*Lepidium Meyenii*		30 mg	*
Muira-Puama	*Ptychopetalum Olacoides*		20 mg	*
Saw Palmetto	*Serenoa Repens*		40 mg	*
Stinging Nettle Leaves	*Urtica Dioica*		40 mg	*
Suma	*Pfaffia Paniculata*		30 mg	*
Turmeric Root	*Curcuma Longa*		10 mg	*

* Recommended Daily Intake has not been established

Other ingredients: Enzymatically processed *Saccharomyces Cerevisiae,* Organic Brown Rice, Vegetarian (HPMC) Capsule.

Suggested use: Serving size or as recommended by your health care professional. Adjust usage according to nutritional lifestyle requirements.

Prosta-Power™ is a 100% Food supplement that is intended to supply nutrients, glandulars, and herbs needed to maintain and support optimal prostate and male health. The prostate secrets seminal fluid that helps enhance the fertility and motility of sperm.

Prosta-Power™ was not designed to be a prostate-cancer fighter. It is intended to provide nutritional support for men interested in natural ways that may improve the health of their prostate and sexual apparatus.

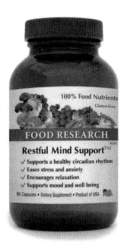

Restful Mind Support™

#680
90 Capsules

√ Supports a healthy circadian rhythm

√ Eases stress and apprehension

√ Encourages relaxation

√ Supports mood and well-being

Supplement Facts
Serving Size 1 Capsule   Servings per Container 90

Amount per Serving		% Daily Value ▼	
Bovine/Ovine Hypothalamus Cytotrophin		5 mg	*
Bovine Ovary Cytotrophin		20 mg	*
Bovine Parotid Cytotrophin		1 mg	*
Bovine Pineal Cytotrophin		5 mg	*
Bovine Pituitary Cytotrophin		5 mg	*
Food Extracted L-Tryptophan	(Grain Extract)	150 mg	*
Wildcrafted Lemon Balm	Melissa Officinalis	214 mg	*

* Recommended Daily Intake has not been established

Other ingredients: Vegetarian (HPMC) Capsule.

Suggested use: Serving size or as recommended by your health care professional. Adjust usage according to nutritional lifestyle requirements.

Restful Mind Support™ is a 100% Food supplement that is intended to supply nutrients, glandulars, and herbs needed to maintain and support optimal feelings of well-being and normal sleep. The pineal gland helps regulate circadian rhythm.

Many people have trouble relaxing and/or sleeping. Some also have anxiety, and sometimes, mood/bipolar, and weight management issues. Insomnia is a common problem. And while there are many causes and hence many interventions for it, the lack of sleep may be pointing to a need for special nutrition.

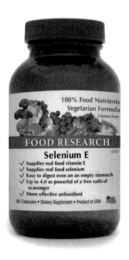

Selenium E™

#707
90 Capsules

√ Supplies real food vitamin E

√ Supplies real food selenium

√ Easy to digest even on an empty stomach

√ Up to 4.0 as powerful of a free radical scavenger

√ More effective antioxidant

Supplement Facts
Serving Size 1 capsule   Servings per container 90

Amount per Serving			% Daily Value ▼	
Vitamin E	(in	250 mg food)	41 mg	279%
Selenium	(in	100 mg food)	100 mcg	180%
Organic Brown Rice	Oryza Sativa		50 mg	*

* Recommended Daily Intake has not been established

Other ingredients: Enzymatically processed *Saccharomyces Cerevisiae*, Vegetarian (HPMC) Capsule.

Suggested use: Serving size or as recommended by your health care professional. Adjust usage according to nutritional lifestyle requirements.

Selenium E™ is a 100% vegan Food supplement that is intended to supply 100% Food vitamin E and selenium.

Vitamin E deficiency has been shown to contribute in progressive peripheral neuropathy and diminished sensory abilities. Selenium often works with vitamin E in the body. Selenium seems to support thyroid hormone production, have antioxidant effects, exists in parts of many enzymes, and supports cardiovascular health.

 Vegetarian Formula

 Halal

 Pareve

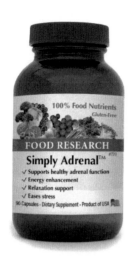

Simply Adrenal™

#720

90 Capsules

√ Supports healthy adrenal
  function

√ Energy enhancement

√ Relaxation support

√ Eases stress

Supplement Facts

Serving Size 1 Capsule   Servings per Container 90

Amount per Serving		% Daily Value ▼
Bovine Adrenal Cytotrophin	200 mg	*

* Recommended Daily Intake has not been established

Other ingredients: Organic Brown Rice, Vegetarian (HPMC) Capsule.

Suggested use: Serving size or as recommended by your health care professional. Adjust usage according to nutritional lifestyle requirements.

Simply Adrenal™ is a 100% Food supplement that is intended to supply nutrients needed to maintain and support optimal adrenal health. **Simply Adrenal™** – This is 200mg per tablet of bovine adrenal tissue. Fauna have most of the same biological materials (like enzymes and other peptides) that humans do.

Adrenal support is often used by people are under stress, fatigued, having difficulty getting up in the morning, who have adrenal stress headaches, or have an abnormal craving for salts. Adrenal tissue is normally taken with meals.

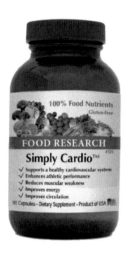

Simply Cardio™

#729

90 Capsules

√ Supports a healthy
  cardiovascular system

√ Enhances athletic performance

√ Reduces muscular weakness

√ Improves energy

√ Improves circulation

Supplement Facts

Serving Size 1 Capsule   Servings per Container 90

Amount per Serving		% Daily Value ▼
Bovine Cardiac Muscle Cytotrophin	200 mg	*

* Recommended Daily Intake has not been established

Other ingredients: Organic Brown Rice, Vegetarian (HPMC) Capsule.

Suggested use: Serving size or as recommended by your health care professional. Adjust usage according to nutritional lifestyle requirements.

Simply Cardio™ is a 100% Food supplement that is intended to supply nutrients needed to maintain and support optimal heart muscle health. The heart pumps blood containing oxygen and other nutrients throughout the body. Bovine heart tissue naturally contains vital heart nutrients like co-enzyme Q10.

Heart tissue has long been used by people interested in supporting healthy heart function.

48

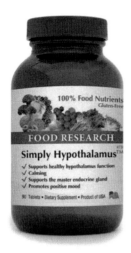

Simply Hypothalamus™

#730
90 Tablets

√ Supports healthy hypothalamus function

√ Calming

√ Supports the master endocrine gland

√ Promotes positive mood

Supplement Facts

Serving Size 1 Tablet   Servings per Container 90

Amount per Serving		% Daily Value▼
Bovine Hypothalamus Cytotrophin	145 mg	*

* Recommended Daily Intake has not been established

Other ingredients: Croscarmellose Sodium *(Digestive Aid)*, Plant Polysaccharide, Silica, Vegetable Oil Extract. Contains No Magnesium Stearate.

Suggested use: Serving size or as recommended by your health care professional. Adjust usage according to nutritional lifestyle requirements.

Simply Hypothalamus™ is a 100% Food supplement that is intended to supply nutrients needed to maintain and support optimal hypothalamus health. The hypothalamus is the body's master endocrine gland. The hypothalamus directly or indirectly controls nearly all the hormonal processes in the body.

The hypothalamus is responsible for the integration of many basic behavioral patterns involving neural and endocrine function.

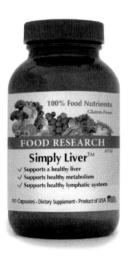

Simply Liver™

#732
90 Capsules

√ Supports a healthy liver

√ Supports healthy metabolism

√ Supports healthy lymphatic system

Supplement Facts

Serving Size 1 Capsule   Servings per Container 90

Amount per Serving		% Daily Value▼
Bovine Liver Cytotrophin	200 mg	*

* Recommended Daily Intake has not been established

Other ingredients: Organic Brown Rice, Vegetarian (HPMC) Capsule.

Suggested use: Serving size or as recommended by your health care professional. Adjust usage according to nutritional lifestyle requirements.

Simply Liver™ is a 100% Food supplement that is intended to supply nutrients needed to maintain and support optimal liver health. The liver is the chemical factory of the body and is also involved in blood sugar regulation.

The liver is the chemical factory of the body and feeding the liver can help when other approaches have not been effective. Historically, bovine liver tissue has long been used by people interested in supporting healthy liver function.

PRODUCTS LABEL INFORMATION

49

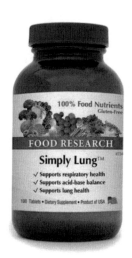

Simply Lung™

#734

100 Tablets

√ Supports respiratory health

√ Supports acid-base balance

√ Supports lung health

Supplement Facts

Serving Size 1 Tablet   Servings per Container 100

Amount per Serving	% Daily Value ▼
Bovine Lung Cytotrophin	200 mg •

* Recommended Daily Intake has not been established

Other ingredients: Croscarmellose Sodium *(Digestive Aid)*, Plant Polysaccharide, Silica, Vegetable Oil Extract. Contains No Magnesium Stearate.

Suggested use: Serving size or as recommended by your health care professional. Adjust usage according to nutritional lifestyle requirements.

Simply Lung™ is a 100% Food supplement that is intended to supply nutrients needed to maintain and support optimal lung health. Bovine lung tissue helps maintain the lungs in a good state of repair to support healthy lung function.

Lungs are necessary for proper respiration. Historically, bovine lung tissue has long been used by people interested in supporting healthy lung function.

Simply Mammary™

#735

100 Tablets

√ Supports breast health

√ Supports female health

Supplement Facts

Serving Size 1 Tablet   Servings per Container 100

Amount per Serving	% Daily Value ▼
Bovine Mammary Cytotrophin	200 mg •

* Recommended Daily Intake has not been established

Other ingredients: Croscarmellose Sodium *(Digestive Aid)*, Plant Polysaccharide, Silica, Vegetable Oil Extract. Contains No Magnesium Stearate.

Suggested use: Serving size or as recommended by your health care professional. Adjust usage according to nutritional lifestyle requirements.

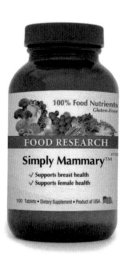

Simply Mammary™ is a 100% Food supplement that is intended to supply nutrients needed to maintain and support optimal breast health. It has been reported that, in theory, the mammary glands can stimulate the ovaries, the hypothalamus, and adrenal glands.

The breasts are involved in lactation, sexual attraction, and sexual response. Historically, bovine mammary tissue has long been used by people interested in supporting healthy breast function.

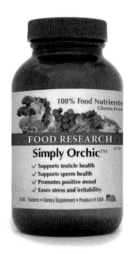

Simply Orchic™

#740
90 Capsules

√ Supports testicle health
√ Supports sperm health
√ Promotes positive mood
√ Eases stress and irritability

Supplement Facts

Serving Size 1 Capsule   Servings per Container 90

Amount per Serving		% Daily Value ▼
Bovine Orchic Cytotrophin	200 mg	*

* Recommended Daily Intake has not been established

Other ingredients: Croscarmellose Sodium *(Digestive Aid)*, Plant Polysaccharide, Silica, Vegetable Oil Extract. Contains No Magnesium Stearate.

Suggested use: Serving size or as recommended by your health care professional. Adjust usage according to nutritional lifestyle requirements.

Simply Orchic™ is a 100% Food supplement that is intended to supply nutrients needed to maintain and support optimal testicle health. Orchic is another name for testicle, a male reproductive gland that produces sperm.

Simply Orchic™ contains many of the substances produced by, or naturally in, those glands including peptides, hormone precursors, and enzymes. Some believe that supplementation with such glands can have a calming and balancing effect on the nervous system.

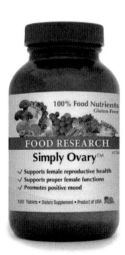

Simply Ovary™

#736
90 Capsules

√ Supports female reproductive health
√ Supports proper female functions
√ Promotes positive mood

Supplement Facts

Serving Size 1 Capsule   Servings per Container 90

Amount per Serving		% Daily Value ▼
Bovine Ovary Cytotrophin	200 mg	*

* Recommended Daily Intake has not been established

Other ingredients: Croscarmellose Sodium *(Digestive Aid)*, Plant Polysaccharide, Silica, Vegetable Oil Extract. Contains No Magnesium Stearate.

Suggested use: Serving size or as recommended by your health care professional. Adjust usage according to nutritional lifestyle requirements.

Simply Ovary™ is a 100% Food supplement that is intended to supply nutrients needed to maintain and support optimal ovary health. Ovaries are female reproductive glands that produce hormones and reproductive cells.

Ovaries are involved various female hormones. Historically, bovine ovary tissue has long been used by women interested in supporting healthy ovarian function. As it has effects that differ from thyroid support, it is often advised to take ovarian tissue before bed.

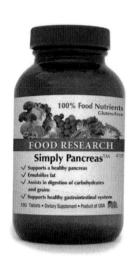

Simply Pancreas™

#737
100 Tablets

√ Supports a healthy pancreas

√ Emulsifies fat

√ Assists in digestion of carbohydrates and grains

√ Supports healthy gastrointestinal system

Supplement Facts
Serving Size 1 Tablet   Servings per Container 100

Amount per Serving	% Daily Value▼

Bovine Pancreas Cytotrophin
   Naturally supplying Amylase, Lipase
   Protease, Trypsin & Chymotrypsin
	200 mg *

* Recommended Daily Intake has not been established

Other ingredients: Croscarmellose Sodium *(Digestive Aid)*, Plant Polysaccharide, Silica, Vegetable Oil Extract. Contains No Magnesium Stearate.

Suggested use: Serving size or as recommended by your health care professional. Adjust usage according to nutritional lifestyle requirements.

Simply Pancreas™ is a 100% Food supplement that is intended to supply nutrients needed to maintain and support optimal pancreas and digestive health. Bovine pancreas tissue helps maintain the pancreas in a good state of repair to support healthy pancreatic function.

The pancreas is instrumental in the regulation of blood sugar and is one of the most important organs related to a healthy digestive system. The pancreas produces trypsin and is operational in intermediate protein metabolism.

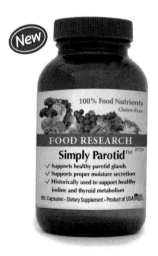

Simply Parotid™

#738
90 Capsules

√ Supports healthy parotid glands

√ Supports proper moisture secretion

√ Historically used to support healthy iodine and thyroid metabolism

Supplement Facts
Serving Size 1 Capsule   Servings per Container 90

Amount per Serving	% Daily Value▼
Bovine Parotid Cytotrophin	200 mg *

* Recommended Daily Intake has not been established

Other ingredients: Organic Brown Rice, Vegetarian (HPMC) Capsule.

Suggested use: Serving size or as recommended by your health care professional. Adjust usage according to nutritional lifestyle requirements.

Simply Parotid™ is a 100% Food supplement that is intended to support healthy parotid glands. The late Dr. Royal Lee also recommended parotid gland extracts for those undescended testicles.

Some people have also found parotid glandulars helpful for detoxification.

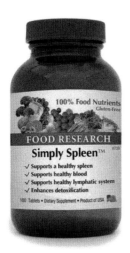

Simply Spleen™

#739

100 Tablets

√ Supports a healthy spleen

√ Supports healthy blood

√ Supports healthy lymphatic system

√ Enhances detoxification

Supplement Facts

Serving Size 1 Tablet   Servings per Container 100

Amount per Serving		% Daily Value ▼
Bovine Spleen Cytotrophin	200 mg	*

* Recommended Daily Intake has not been established

Other ingredients: Croscarmellose Sodium *(Digestive Aid)*, Plant Polysaccharide, Silica, Vegetable Oil Extract. Contains No Magnesium Stearate.

Suggested use: Serving size or as recommended by your health care professional. Adjust usage according to nutritional lifestyle requirements.

Simply Spleen™ is a 100% Food supplement that is intended to supply nutrients needed to maintain and support optimal spleen health. Bovine spleen tissue helps maintain the spleen tissues in a good state of repair to support healthy spleen function.

Spleen is the body's largest lymphatic organ and is involved with detoxification. Historically, bovine spleen tissue has long been used by people interested in supporting healthy spleen function.

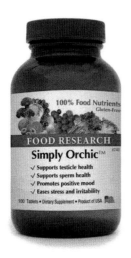

Simply Thymus™

#742

100 Tablets

√ Enhanced immune health

√ Supports skin health

√ Supports a healthy thymus gland

Supplement Facts

Serving Size 1 Tablet   Servings per Container 100

Amount per Serving		% Daily Value ▼
Bovine Thymus Cytotrophin	200 mg	*

* Recommended Daily Intake has not been established

Other ingredients: Croscarmellose Sodium *(Digestive Aid)*, Plant Polysaccharide, Silica, Vegetable Oil Extract. Contains No Magnesium Stearate.

Suggested use: Serving size or as recommended by your health care professional. Adjust usage according to nutritional lifestyle requirements.

Simply Thymus™ is a 100% Food supplement that is intended to supply nutrients needed to maintain and support optimal thymus and immune system health. Bovine thymus tissue helps maintain the thymus gland in a good state of repair to support healthy thymus function.

Bovine thymus tissue is often used for immune system support. Historically, bovine thymus tissue has long been used by people interested in supporting healthy thymus function.

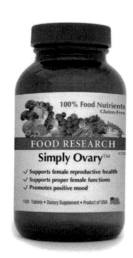

Simply Thyroid™

#746

100 Tablets

√ Supports a healthy thyroid

√ Enhances energy

√ Supports proper metabolism

√ Mood support

Supplement Facts

Serving Size 1 Tablet   Servings per Container 100

Amount per Serving		% Daily Value▼
Bovine Thyroid Cytotrophin	200 mg	*

* Recommended Daily Intake has not been established

Other ingredients: Croscarmellose Sodium *(Digestive Aid)*, Plant Polysaccharide, Silica, Vegetable Oil Extract. Contains No Magnesium Stearate.

Suggested use: Serving size or as recommended by your health care professional. Adjust usage according to nutritional lifestyle requirements.

Simply Thyroid™ is a 200mg per tablet of bovine thyroid tissue *(Note: bovine thyroid glands are thyroxine-free, thus do not result in a shutting down of the thyroid gland when taken).* Bovine thyroid tissue helps maintain thyroid tissues in a good state of repair to support healthy thyroid function.

The thyroid produces hormones that impact metabolism and calcium retention. Thyroid tissue is used by people with metabolism issues. Historically, bovine thyroid tissue has long been used by people interested in supporting healthy thyroid function.

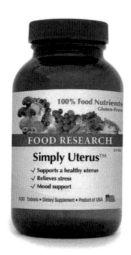

Simply Uterus™

#748

100 Tablets

√ Supports a healthy uterus

√ Relieves stress

√ Mood support

Supplement Facts

Serving Size 1 Tablet   Servings per Container 100

Amount per Serving		% Daily Value▼
Bovine Uterus Cytotrophin	200 mg	*

* Recommended Daily Intake has not been established

Other ingredients: Croscarmellose Sodium *(Digestive Aid)*, Plant Polysaccharide, Silica, Vegetable Oil Extract. Contains No Magnesium Stearate.

Suggested use: Serving size or as recommended by your health care professional. Adjust usage according to nutritional lifestyle requirements.

Simply Uterus™ is a 200mg per tablet of bovine uterine tissue. Bovine uterus tissue has long been advised to improve the integrity of uterus cells and to assist with a whole range of menstrual and menopausal concerns. Bovine uterus tissue helps maintain uterine tissues in a good state of repair to support healthy uterine function.

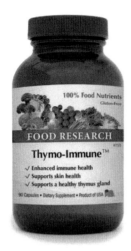

Thymo-Immune™

#750

90 Capsules

√ Enhanced immune health

√ Supports skin health

√ Supports a healthy thymus gland

Other ingredients: Vegetarian (HPMC) Capsule.

Suggested use: Serving size or as recommended by your health care professional. Adjust usage according to nutritional lifestyle requirements.

Not Recommended During Pregnancy.

Thymo-Immune™ is a 100% Food supplement that is intended to supply nutrients needed to maintain and support optimal thymus and immune system health. Bovine thymus tissue helps maintain the thymus gland in a good state of repair to support healthy thymus function.

Thymo-Immune™ contains acerola cherry which is one of the most vitamin C dense foods. Vitamin C, carrot root and garlic provide support for a healthy immune system.

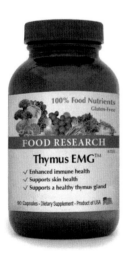

Thymus EMG™

#755

90 Capsules

√ Enhanced immune health

√ Supports skin health

√ Supports a healthy thymus gland

Other ingredients: Organic Brown Rice, Vegetarian (HPMC) Capsule.

Suggested use: Serving size or as recommended by your health care professional. Adjust usage according to nutritional lifestyle requirements.

Thymus EMG™ is a 100% Food supplement that is intended to supply nutrients needed to maintain and support optimal thymus and immune system health. Bovine thymus tissue helps maintain the thymus gland in a good state of repair to support healthy thymus function.

Thymus EMG™ contains an Enzomorphogen extract which are uniquely derived in order to support cellular health.

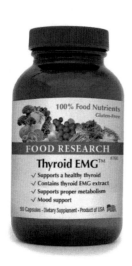

Thyroid EMG™

#760
90 Capsules

√ Supports a healthy thyroid

√ Contains thyroid EMG extract

√ Supports proper metabolism

√ Mood support

Supplement Facts
Serving Size 1 Capsule Servings per Container 90

Amount per Serving		% Daily Value▼	
Bovine Thyroid Cytotrophin		30 mg	*
(Processed to Substantially Remove Thyroxine)			
Collinsonia Root	Collinsonia Canadensis	30 mg	*
Bovine Chymotrypsin		0.016 mg	*
Bovine Trypsin		0.007 mg	*

* Recommended Daily Intake has not been established

Other ingredients: Organic Brown Rice, Vegetarian (HPMC) Capsule.

Suggested use: Serving size or as recommended by your health care professional. Adjust usage according to nutritional lifestyle requirements.

Thyroid EMG™ is a 100% Food supplement product for those desiring mild nutritional support for a healthy thyroid.

Thyroid EMG™ contains an Enzomorphogen extract which are uniquely derived in order to support cellular health.

All FOOD RESEARCH Products are 100% Food Nutrients!

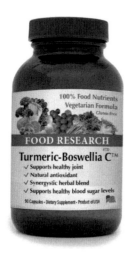

Turmeric-Boswellia C™

#770
90 Capsules

√ Supports healthy joints

√ Natural antioxidant

√ Synergystic herbal blend

√ Supports healthy blood sugar levels

Supplement Facts
Serving Size 1 Capsule   Servings per Container 90

Amount per Serving		% Daily Value▼	
Vitamin C	(in 36 mg food)	9 mg	10%
Acerola Cherry	Malpighia Glabra	36 mg	*
Boswellia Gum	Boswellia Serrata	125 mg	*
Fenugreek	Trigonella Foenum-Graecum	100 mg	*
Ginger Rhizome	Zingiber Officinale	39 mg	*
Turmeric Rhizome	Curcuma Longa	200 mg	*

* Recommended Daily Intake has not been established

Other ingredients: Vegetarian (HPMC) Capsule.

Suggested use: Serving size or as recommended by your health care professional. Adjust usage according to nutritional lifestyle requirements.

Turmeric-Boswellia C™ is a synergystic blend of herbs which also supplies 100% Food vitamin C.

Turmeric-Boswellia C™ supplies herbs which have traditionally been used to support joint health and comfort. Some of the herbs also can support healthy blood sugar levels.

 Vegetarian Formula

 Halal

 Pareve

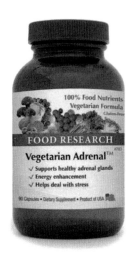

Vegetarian Adrenal™

#783
90 Capsules

√ Supports healthy adrenal glands

√ Energy enhancement

√ Helps deal with stress

Supplement Facts
Serving Size 3 Capsules   Servings per Container 30

Amount per Serving				% Daily Value ▼
Vitamin C	(in	600 mg food)	150 mg	166%
Vitamin B-6	(in	1.2 mg food)	.24 mg	14%
Folate (Vitamin B-9)	(in	.8 mg food)	8 mcg DFE	2%
Vitamin B-12 – Methylated	(in	.12 mg food)	.6 mcg	25%
Pantothenate (Vitamin B-5)	(in	20 mg food)	5 mg	100%
Acerola Cherry	Malpighia Glabra		600 mg	*
Carob Pod	Ceratonia Siliqua		20 mg	*
Food Extracted L-Serine	(Plant Source)		180 mg	*
Food Extracted L-Tyrosine	(Plant Source)		60 mg	*
Organic Brown Rice	Oryza Sativa		30 mg	*
Wildcrafted Ashwagandha	Withania Somnifera		60 mg	*
Wildcrafted Kelp Thallus	Ascophyllum Nodosum		30 mg	*
Wildcrafted Tomato (Powder)	Lycopersicum Esculentum		60 mg	*

* Recommended Daily Intake has not been established

Other ingredients: Enzymatically Processed *Saccharomyces Cerevisiae*, Vegetarian (HPMC) Capsule.

Suggested use: Serving size or as recommended by your health care professional. Adjust usage according to nutritional lifestyle requirements.

 Vegetarian Formula

 Halal   Pareve

Vegetarian Adrenal™ is a 100% vegan Food supplement intended to nutritionally support the adrenal glands and help support biochemical imbalances associated with cortisol production. The adrenal glands play a role in energy, stress, mood, and even pain control. The adrenal glands have probably the greatest store of vitamin C in the body.

Vegetarian Adrenal™ is basically Food intended for the adrenal glands. If additional endocrine support is indicated, consider adding Vegetarian Thyro or Vegetarian Tyrosine.

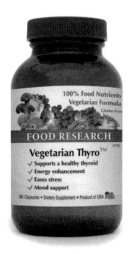

Vegetarian Thyro™

#796
90 Capsules

√ Supports a healthy thyroid

√ Energy enhancement

√ Eases stress

√ Mood support

Supplement Facts
Serving Size 1 Capsule   Servings per Container 90

Amount per Serving				% Daily Value ▼
Vitamin B-6	(in	1.2 mg food)	.24 mg	14%
Folate (Vitamin B-9)	(in	.8 mg food)	8 mcg DFE	2%
Vitamin B-12 – Methylated	(in	.12 mg food)	.60 mcg	25%
Zinc	(in	12.5 mg food)	625 mcg	5%
Dong Quai Root	Angelica Sinensis		55 mg	*
Food Extracted L-Tyrosine	(Plant Source)		150 mg	*
Organic Carrot Root	Daucus Carota		25 mg	*
Wildcrafted Burdock Root	Articum Lappa		55 mg	*
Wildcrafted Icelandic Moss	Cetraria Islandica		37 mg	*
Wildcrafted Kelp Thallus	Ascophyllum Nodesum		62 mg	*

* Recommended Daily Intake has not been established

Other ingredients: Enzymatically Processed *Saccharomyces Cerevisiae*, Vegetarian (HPMC) Capsule.

Suggested use: Serving size or as recommended by your health care professional. Adjust usage according to nutritional lifestyle requirements.

Not Recommended During Pregnancy.

 Vegetarian Formula

 Halal   Pareve

Vegetarian Thyro™ is a 100% vegan Food supplement intended to nutritionally support the thyroid and improve metabolism. Vegetarian Thyro is basically Food intended for the thyroid gland.

The thyroid is responsible for hormones that affect mood, improve circulation, increase metabolism, retain calcium, affect cardiovascular health, and improve tolerance to temperature fluctuations.

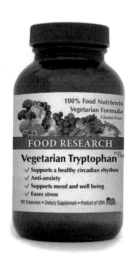

Vegetarian Tryptophan™

#797
90 Capsules

√ Supports a healthy circadian rhythm

√ Anti-anxiety

√ Supports mood and well-being

√ Eases stress

Supplement Facts		
Serving Size 1 Capsule	Servings per Container 90	
Amount per Serving		**% Daily Value▼**
Food Extracted L-Tryptophan (From Vegetables)	500 mg	*
* Recommended Daily Intake has not been established		

Other ingredients: Vegetarian (HPMC) Capsule.

Suggested use: Serving size or as recommended by your health care professional. Adjust usage according to nutritional lifestyle requirements.

Vegetarian Tryptophan™ is a 100% vegetarian Food supplement that supplies tryptophan.

"L-tryptophan is an essential amino acid, which must be consumed from food since the body cannot make it using other amino acids. It is present in virtually all plant and animal proteins. It is primarily the serotonin that does all the wonderful things attributed to L-tryptophan."

 Vegetarian Formula

 Halal Pareve

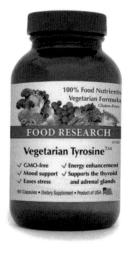

Vegetarian Tyrosine™

#798
90 Capsules

√ GMO-free

√ Mood support

√ Eases stress

√ Energy enhancement

√ Supports the thyroid and adrenal glands

Supplement Facts			
Serving Size 1 Capsule		Servings per Container 90	
Amount per Serving			**% Daily Value▼**
Food Extracted L-Tyrosine	(Vegan GMO-Free)	480 mg	*
Pumpkin Seeds	Cucurbita Maxima	20 mg	*
* Recommended Daily Intake has not been established			

Other ingredients: Vegetarian (HPMC) Capsule.

Suggested use: Serving size or as recommended by your health care professional. Adjust usage according to nutritional lifestyle requirements.

Vegetarian Tyrosine™ is a 100% vegan Food supplement that is intended to supply nutrients needed to provide high quality vegan tyrosine and support factors. Tyrosine is an amino acid that some have trouble producing and is used by the thyroid and adrenal glands.

Vegetarian Tyrosine™ naturally contains carbohydrates, lipids, proteins (including essential amino acids) — all the nutrients shown above are contained in beans or a fermented bean extract.

 Vegetarian Formula

 Halal Pareve

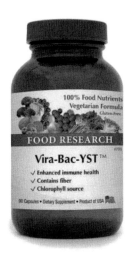

Vira-Bac-YST™

#799

90 Capsules

√ Enhanced immune health

√ Contains fiber

√ Chlorophyll source

Supplement Facts		
Serving Size 1 Capsule Servings per Container 90		
Amount per Serving		**% Daily Value ▼**
Buckwheat Leaf	Fagopyrum Esculentum	75 mg	*
Olive Leaf Extract	Olea Europaea	75 mg	*
Wildcrafted Beet Root	Beta Vulgaris	80 mg	*
Wildcrafted Oregano Leaf	Origanum Vulgare	100 mg	*

* Recommended Daily Intake has not been established

Other ingredients: Vegetarian (HPMC) Capsule.

Suggested use: Serving size or as recommended by your health care professional. Adjust usage according to nutritional lifestyle requirements.

Vira-Bac-YST™ is a vegan 100% food supplement that is intended to support a healthy immune and digestive system. It contains herbs such as Wild Oregano. It enhances immune health, contains fiber, and is a Chlorophyll source.

Vira-Bac-YST™ naturally contains carbohydrates, lipids, proteins (including essential amino acids), as found in Buckwheat Leaf, Olive Leaf Concentrate, and Wild Oregano.

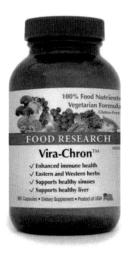

Vira-Chron™

#800

90 Capsules

√ Enhanced immune health

√ Eastern and Western herbs

√ Supports healthy sinuses

√ Supports healthy liver

Supplement Facts		
Serving Size 1 Capsule Servings per Container 90		
Amount per Serving		**% Daily Value ▼**
Angelica Root	Angelica Sinensis	23 mg	*
Bupleurum Root	Bupleurum Chinense	23 mg	*
Chaste Tree Berry	Vitex Agnus Castus	23 mg	*
Coptis Root	Coptis Chinensis	40 mg	*
Forsythia Root	Forsythia Suspensa	23 mg	*
Gardenia Fruit	Gardenia Jasminoides	40 mg	*
Lonicera Flower	Jin Yin Hua	40 mg	*
Magnolia Bark	Xin Yi Hua	23 mg	*
Olive Leaf Extract	Oleo Europeae	23 mg	*
Phellodendron Bark	Huang Bai	40 mg	*
Red Peony Root	Paeonia Lactiflora	23 mg	*
Wildcrafted Glycyrrhiza	Gan Cao	10 mg	*
Wildcrafted Nettle Leaf	Urtica Dioica	23 mg	*
Wildcrafted Oregano Leaf	Organum Vulgare	23 mg	*
Xanthium Fruit	Xanthium Sibiricum	23 mg	*

* Recommended Daily Intake has not been established

Other ingredients: Vegetarian (HPMC) Capsule.

Suggested use: Serving size or as recommended by your health care professional. Adjust usage according to nutritional lifestyle requirements.

Vira-Chron™ is a 100% vegetarian Food supplement that is intended to supply nutrients needed to maintain and support optimal immune system health.

Vira-Chron™ enhances immune health, contains a variety of Western and Eastern (Chinese) herbs that have historically, as well as recently, been used to support the immune system. It supports a healthy liver and healthy sinuses. It is also taken by some to support digestive system health when imbalances there are encountered.

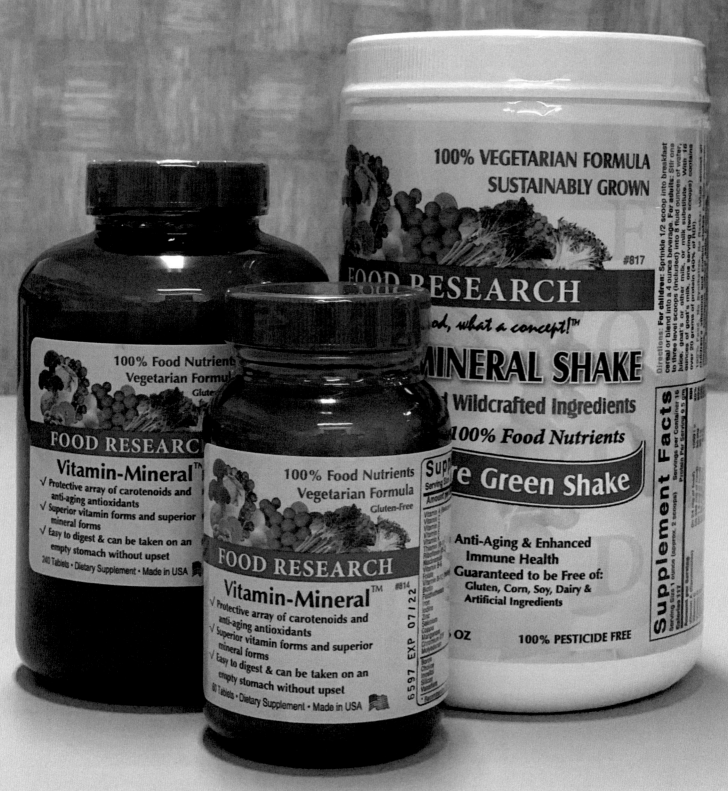

100% VEGETARIAN FORMULA
SUSTAINABLY GROWN

#817

FOOD RESEARCH

...od, what a concept!™

MINERAL SHAKE

Wildcrafted Ingredients

100% Food Nutrients

re Green Shake

Anti-Aging & Enhanced
Immune Health
Guaranteed to be Free of:
Gluten, Corn, Soy, Dairy &
Artificial Ingredients

OZ   100% PESTICIDE FREE

100% Food Nutrients
Vegetarian Formula
Glut

FOOD RESEARCH

Vitamin-Mineral™

√ Protective array of carotenoids and
  anti-aging antioxidants
√ Superior vitamin forms and superior
  mineral forms
√ Easy to digest & can be taken on an
  empty stomach without upset

240 Tablets • Dietary Supplement • Made in USA

100% Food Nutrients
Vegetarian Formula
Gluten-Free

FOOD RESEARCH

Vitamin-Mineral™ #814

√ Protective array of carotenoids and
  anti-aging antioxidants
√ Superior vitamin forms and superior
  mineral forms
√ Easy to digest & can be taken on an
  empty stomach without upset

80 Tablets • Dietary Supplement • Made in USA

6597 EXP 07/22

*FOOD Vitamins and Minerals
ARE Better!*

Vitamin & Mineral Shake™

#817

16 Scoops

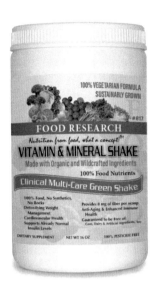

√ 100% Food, No Synthetics, No Rocks

√ Detoxifying Weight Management

√ Cardiovascular Health

√ Supports Already Normal Insulin Levels

√ Anti-Aging & Enhanced Immune Health

√ Guaranteed to be Free of: Gluten, Corn, Soy, Dairy & Artificial Ingredients

The foods in **Vitamin & Mineral Shake™** naturally supply Calcium, Magnesium, Phosphorus, and Potassium, as well as Carbohydrates, Lipids, Monosaccharides (including all considered essential), Proteins (including all ten essential amino acids), Superoxide Dismutase, and Trace Minerals as found in enzymatically processed *Saccharomyces Cerevisiae*, Acerola Cherries, Whole Oranges, Carrots, Broccoli, Cabbage, and Rice—all vitamins and minerals shown above are contained in these foods.

Food Wildcrafted and Organic, **Vitamin-Mineral™** is a food multi-vitamin, multi-mineral formula (and not a synthetic isolate). **Vitamin-Mineral™** does not contain any synthetic USP nutrients, only contains foods, food complexes, and food concentrates. Studies indicate that Food nutrients ARE better than isolated USP nutrients and MAY BE better absorbed, retained, and utilized than USP nutrients.

Supplement Facts

Serving Size 1 ounce (approx. 1 scoop) — Servings per Container 16

Calories 117 — Protein Per Serving 9.5 gm

Amount per Serving				RDI
Vitamin A (Betacarotene)	(in	24 mg food)	360 rae	40%
Vitamin C	(in	240 mg food)	60 mg	66%
Vitamin D	(in	.2 mg food)	200 i.u.	25%
Vitamin E	(in	24 mg food)	6 i.u.	30%
Vitamin K	(in	24 mg food)	24 mcg	20%
Vitamin B1	(in	2.4 mg food)	600 mcg	50%
Vitamin B2	(in	6 mg food)	600 mcg	46%
Niacinamide	(in	24 mg food)	6 mg NE	37%
Vitamin B6	(in	3 mg food)	600 mcg	35%
Folate	(in	8.4 mg food)	80 mcg DFE	20%
Vitamin B12 (Methylated)	(in	1 mg food)	4.8 mcg	200%
Biotin	(in	12 mg food)	60 mcg	200%
Pantothenate	(in	9 mg food)	2.4 mg	48%
Iodine	(in	30 mg food)	30 mcg	20%
Zinc	(in	60 mg food)	3 mg	27%
Selenium	(in	14 mg food)	14 mcg	25%
Copper	(in	4 mg food)	200 mcg	22%
Manganese	(in	12 mg food)	600 mcg	26%
Chromium GTF	(in	12 mg food)	24 mcg	68%
Molybdenum	(in	7.5 mg food)	15 mcg	33%
Acid-Stabilized Enzyme Blend (Amylase, Cellulase, Lactase, Lipase, Maltase, Protease I & II)			16 mg	*
Boron	(in	4 mg food)	40 mcg	*
Non-dairy Acidophilus (Probiotic)			100,000 units	*
Silicon	(in	30 mg food)	300 mcg	*

Acerola Cherry (5% Vitamin C)	Malpighia Glabra	240 mg	*
Carrots (Herbicide/Pesticide Free)	Darcus Carota	24 mg	*
Organic Alfalfa Leaf	Medicago Sativa	4 mg	*
Organic Barley Grass	Hordeum Vulgare	32 mg	*
Organic Brown Rice	Oryza Sativa	4120 mg	*
Organic Celery Seed	Apium Graveolens	16 mg	*
Organic Cinnamon Bark	Cinnamomum Cassia	860 mg	*
Organic Grapes	Vitis Vinifera	360 mg	*
Organic Hemp	Cannabis Sativa	18940 mg	*
Organic Parsley Leaf	Petroselinum Crispum	16 mg	*
Organic Peppermint	Mentha Piperita	1000 mg	*
Organic Spinach Leaf	Spinacia Oleracea	32 mg	*
Organic Stevia	Stevia Rebaudiana	1600 mg	*
Organic Vanilla	Vanilla Planifolia	32 mg	*
Organic Watercress	Nasturtium Officinale	8 mg	*
Organic Wheatgrass	Triticum Aestivum	32 mg	*
Wildcrafted Spirulina	Spirulina spp	1630 mg	*

* Recommended Daily Intake has not been established

Other ingredients: Enzymatically processed *Saccharomyces Cerevisiae*.

Suggested use: Serving size or as recommended by your health care professional. Adjust usage according to nutritional lifestyle requirements.

Food Research Guarantee: The ingredients in this product are certified organic and/or are grown purely and not chemically. Guaranteed to contain NO gluten, corn, soy, dairy, preservatives, artificial sweeteners, inorganic minerals, or synthetic vitamins.

 Vegetarian Formula

 Halal   Pareve

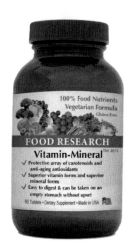

Vitamin-Mineral™

#814 – Small/90T
#815 – Large/270T

√ Protective array of carotenoids and anti–aging antioxidants

√ Superior vitamin forms and superior mineral forms

√ Easy to digest & can be taken on an empty stomach without upset

Supplement Facts
Serving Size 3 Tablets   Servings per Container 30

Amount per Serving			% Daily Value ▼	
Vitamin A (Betacarotene)	(in	60 mg food)	900 rae	100%
Vitamin C	(in	540 mg food)	135 mg	150%
Vitamin D	(in	.80 mg food)	800 i.u.	100%
Vitamin E	(in	120 mg food)	30 mg	200%
Vitamin K	(in	6 mg food)	60 mcg	50%
Thiamin (Vitamin B-1)	(in	10 mg food)	2.4 mg	200%
Riboflavin (Vitamin B-2)	(in	26 mg food)	2.6 mg	200%
Niacinamide (Vitamin B-3)	(in	112 mg food)	28 mg NE	175%
Vitamin B-6	(in	15 mg food)	3 mg	176%
Folate (Vitamin B-9)	(in	40 mg food)	400 mcg DFE	100%
Vitamin B-12 – Methylated	(in	1.92 mg food)	9.6 mcg	400%
Biotin (Vitamin B-7)	(in	12 mg food)	60 mcg	200%
Panthothenate (Vitamin B-5)	(in	40 mg food)	10 mg	200%
Iron	(in	180 mg food)	9 mg	50%
Iodine	(in	10 mg food)	150 mcg	100%
Zinc	(in	220 mg food)	11 mg	100%
Selenium	(in	55 mg food)	55 mcg	100%
Copper	(in	90 mg food)	.9 mg	100%
Manganese	(in	46 mg food)	2.3 mg	100%
Chromium GTF	(in	22.5 mg food)	45 mcg	150%
Molybdenum	(in	22.5 mg food)	45 mcg	100%
Choline	(in	220 mg food)	55 mg	10%
Boron	(in	8 mg food)	75 mcg	•
Inositol	(in	8 mg food)	2 mg	•
Silicon	(in	150 mg food)	1500 mcg	•
Vanadium	(in	25 mg food)	25 mcg	•

* Recommended Daily Intake has not been established

Other ingredients: Enzymatically processed *Saccharomyces Cerevisiae*, Vegetable Oil Extract, Vegetarian Coating.

Suggested use: Serving size or as recommended by your health care professional. Adjust usage according to nutritional lifestyle requirements.

 Halal   Pareve

Vitamin-Mineral™ is a 100% vegetarian Food supplement that is the best multi-vitamin, multi-mineral product available anywhere. Unlike some other claimed "whole food" multi-formulas, it does not contain ANY isolate USP nutrients, plus it contains the RDI amount of the more costly food nutrients such as chromium GTF.

All nutrients are contained in the following foods: Acerola Cherry, Alfalfa, Organic Brown Rice, Carrots, Enzymatically processed *Saccharomyces Cerevisiae* and Oranges.

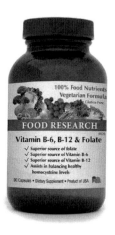

Vitamin B-6, B-12 & Folate™

#826

90 Capsules

√ Superior source of folate

√ Superior source of Vitamin B-6

√ Superior source of Vitamin B-12

√ Assits in balancing healthy Homocysteine levels

Supplement Facts
Serving Size 1 Capsule   Servings per Container 90

Amount per Serving		% Daily Value ▼	
Vitamin B-6	(in 125 mg food)	25 mg	1470%
Folate (Vitamin B-9)	(in 80 mg food)	800 mcg DFE	200%
Vitamin B-12 – Methylated	(in 6 mg food)	30 mcg	1250%
Wildcrafted Beet Root	*Beta Vulgaris*	180 mg	*

* Recommended Daily Intake has not been established

Other ingredients: Enzymatically Processed *Saccharomyces Cerevisiae*, Vegetarian (HPMC) Capsule.

Suggested use: Serving size or as recommended by your health care professional. Adjust usage according to nutritional lifestyle requirements.

 Halal   Pareve

Vitamin B6, B12, & Folate™ is a 100% vegan Food supplement that is intended to supply nutrients needed to provide high quality 100% Food vitamins B6, B12 and B9 (folate). Vitamins B6, B12, and B9 support healthy blood. B12 is essential for myelin synthesis and central nervous system function.

Unlike most so-called "natural" supplements, this product does not contain any folic acid, which is a sythetic from of vitamin B-9 and is dangerous.

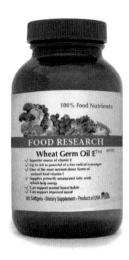

Wheat Germ Oil E™

#870

90 Softgels

√ Superior source of vitamin E

√ Up to 4.0 as powerful of a free radical scavenger

√ One of the most nutrient-dense forms of vitamin E available anywhere

√ Supplies primarily unsaturated fatty acids which help energy

Supplement Facts

Serving Size 1 Softgel   Servings per Container 90

Amount per Serving	% Daily Value ▼
Wheat Germ Oil	1130 mg	*

* Recommended Daily Intake has not been established

Other ingredients: Gelatin (Bovine Lime Bone), Glycerine, Water.

Suggested use: Serving size or as recommended by your health care professional. Adjust usage according to nutritional lifestyle requirements.

√ Can support normal bowel habits

√ Can support improved mood

Wheat Germ Oil E™ is a 100% Food supplement that is intended to supply nutrients needed to provide high quality 100% Food vitamin E.

Wheat Germ Oil E™ is one of the most naturally concentrated food forms of vitamin E. Wheat germ oil naturally also contains octacosonal and has been used by some intertested in better athletic performance and mood support.

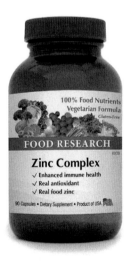

Zinc Complex™

#909

90 Capsules

√ Enhanced immune health

√ Real antioxidant

√ Real food zinc

Supplement Facts

Serving Size 1 Capsule   Servings per Container 90

Amount per Serving		% Daily Value ▼
Zinc	(in 375 mg food)	18.75 mg	170%
Pumpkin Seed	*Cucurbita Pepo*	25 mg	*

* Recommended Daily Intake has not been established

Other ingredients: Enzymatically Processed *Saccharomyces Cerevisiae,* Vegetarian (HPMC) Capsule.

Suggested use: Serving size or as recommended by your health care professional. Adjust usage according to nutritional lifestyle requirements.

Zinc Complex™ is a 100% vegetarian Food supplement that is intended to supply nutrients needed to provide high quality 100% Food organic zinc (as opposed to inorganic mineral salt forms).

Zinc Complex™ contains naturally occurring carbohydrates, lipids, proteins (including all ten essential amino acids), superoxide dismutase, and truly organic bioflavonoids as found in enzymatically processed *Saccharomyces Cervisiae* and organic pumpkin seeds *Cucurbita pepo*— all the nutrients shown above are contained in these foods.

 Vegetarian Formula
 GLUTEN FREE

 Halal
 Pareve

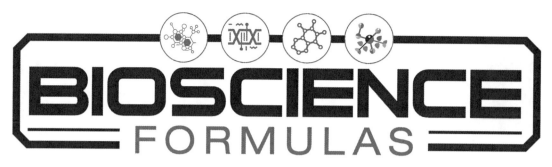

BIOSCIENCE FORMULAS

Bioscience Formulas differs from Food Research brand in that it may claim nutrients from non-food sources including bones and a broader form of glandular sources.

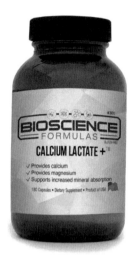

CALCIUM LACTATE +™

BF #301
180 Capsules

√ Provides calcium

√ Provides magnesium

√ Supports increased mineral absorption

SUPPLEMENT FACTS		
Serving size 4 Capsules	Serving per Container 45	
Amount per Serving	**% Daily Value** ▼	
Calcium (as Lactate)	243 mg	19%
Magnesium (as Citrate)	55 mg	13%
Betain HCL	300 mg	*
Bovine Spleen	300 mg	*
Organic Peppermint Leaf Mentha Piperita	150 mg	*
* Recommended Daily Intake has not been established		

Other ingredients: Vegetarian Capsule.

Suggested use: Serving size or as recommended by your health care professional. Adjust usage according to nutritional lifestyle requirements.

Calcium Lactate + ™ is intended for those who would like mineral salt calcium and magnesium support. Calcium supports healthy bones, and is also involved with muscle contractions, nerve conduction, and cell membranes.

DENTO-GUMS™

BF #302
180 Tablets

√ Chewable calcium

√ Supports healthy bones and teeth

√ Supports healthy gums

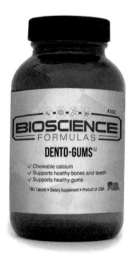

SUPPLEMENT FACTS		
Serving size 1 Tablet Serving per Container 180		
Amount per Serving	**% Daily Value** ▼	
Vitamin C (in Acerola Cherry)	3 mg	3%
Calcium (in Bovine Bone)	75 mg	6%
Acerola Cherry Malpighia Glabra	12 mg	*
Bovine Adrenal	10 mg	*
Bovine Bone Marrow	50 mg	*
Bovine Bone Meal	280 mg	*
Bovine Cartilage	30 mg	*
Bovine Spleen	10 mg	*
Licorice Root Glycyrrhiza Glabra	20 mg	*
Neem Leaf Extract Powder Azadirachta Indica	20 mg	*
Organic Carrot Root Daucus Carrota	30 mg	*
Organic Rice Bran Oryza Sativa	8 mg	*
Wild Yam Root Dioscorea Villosa	20 mg	*
Wheat Germ (Defatted) Triticum Aestivum	20 mg	*
* Recommended Daily Intake has not been established		

Other ingredients: Croscarmellose Sodium (Digestive Aid), Vegetable Oil Extract, Honey, Organic Strawberry Powder, Silica. Contains No Magnesium Stearate.

Suggested use: Serving size or as recommended by your health care professional. Adjust usage according to nutritional lifestyle requirements.

Dento-Gums™ provides nutrients found in healthy teeth, bones, and gums. For better absorbality in the mouth, chewing the product before swallowing is recommended.

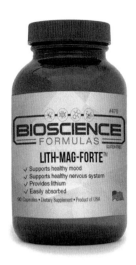

LITH-MAG-FORTE™

BF #470

90 Capsules

√ Supports healthy mood
√ Supports healthy nervous system
√ Provides lithium

SUPPLEMENT FACTS

Serving size 1 Capsule | Serving per Container 90

Amount per Serving		% Daily Value ▼
Magnesium *(Amino Acid Chelate)*		52 mg	12.4%
Lithium *(Lithium Orotate)*		2 mg	*
Lion's Mane	*Hericium Erinaceus*	100 mg	*
Collinsonia Root	*Collinsonia Canadensis*	56 mg	*

* Recommended Daily Intake has not been established

Other ingredients: Vegetarian (HPMC) Capsule

Suggested use: Serving size or as recommended by your health care professional. Adjust usage according to nutritional lifestyle requirements.

Lith-Mag-Forte™ is used to support a healthy mood. It upregulates neurotrophins, including brain-derived neurotrophic factor (BDNF), nerve growth factor, neurotrophin-3 (NT3), as well as receptors to these growth factors in the brain.

► **Collinsonia Root** has tonic effects. The tonic effects within the bowels help maintain a state of calm throughout the body.

► **Lion's Mane** naturally contains substances that often helps mood and the body's ability to hand stress.

► **Lithium** stimulates proliferation of stem cells, including bone marrow and neural stem cells in the subventricular zone, striatum and forebrain. **Lithium** increases brain concentrations of the neuronal markers n-acetyl-aspartate and myoinositol.

► **Magnesium** is an essential mineral that "is involved in over 300 metabolic reactions" and relaxes muscles. Some people report that Magnesium helps with mood.

Food Research Products Test Kit

Available!

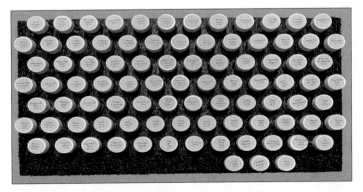

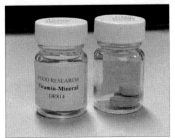

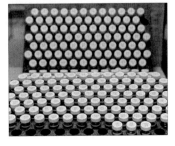

Doctors' Research is pleased to announce that we now have a **FOOD RESEARCH** Test Kit available for you. We understand that each individual has unique health needs and that not all supplements will work the same for everyone.

Because of this, we have assembled a convenient test kit that includes our entire line of **FOOD RESEARCH** and **BIOSCIENCE FORMULAS** supplements.

We trust that our test kit will provide you with an efficient way to test and recommend the best supplements for your clients based on their individual needs.

Doctors' Research Support Literature and Educational Items

A great deal of technical support literature on our line of Food products is available at our Website (www.doctorsresearch.com). There are also individual technical bulletins available on each of our Food products.

In addition, there are some educational items that we have found seem to help support many of the benefits of Food vitamin and mineral supplements. These support materials can help compliance and demonstrate to your clients that there are many differences between Food and non-food supplements. They can help your clients better understand the benefits of Food vitamins and minerals, as well as how unnatural the so-called 'natural' vitamin and mineral supplements are that they are currently taking.

It is an economic fact that it costs at least ten times as much to attract a new client, than it does to retain the ones you have. Our support literature is designed to help you retain your existing clients, while also (in the case of the Food Brochure) helping you attract new clients.

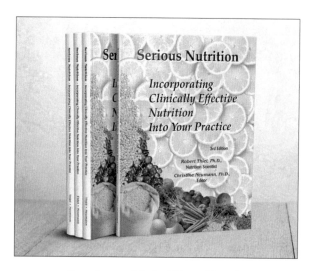

Serious Nutrition Book

Incorporating Clinically Effective Nutrition into Your Practice - This book, written by Robert Thiel, Ph.D., Board-Certified Naturopath and Nutrition Scientist, is a comprehensive book on the use of clinically-effective nutrition. It discusses multiple disease conditions, various types of assessment, provides forms, diets, and more. It contains information on individual nutrients, including individual vitamins, minerals, herbs, glandulars, and amino acids.

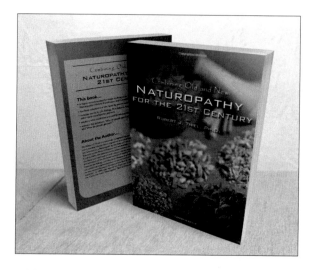

Naturopathy for the 21st Century

Combining Old and New: Naturopathy for the 21st Century - This book, written by Robert Thiel, Ph.D., Board-Certified Naturopath, is the most comprehensive book currently in print on naturopathy. It explains how people get sick, how people get well, as well as natural interventions often used by naturopaths. It contains writings from many current and historical naturopaths, and even explains advantages of natural Food vitamins and minerals over their synthetic counterparts. In addition to naturopathic schools, Ohio University and Portland State University have used it as a textbook.

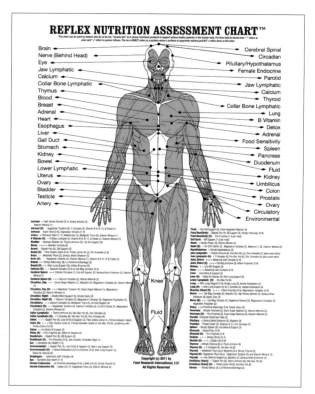

Muscle Testing Wall Chart

This international, colorized, chart, titled Reflex Nutrition Assessment, is intended for the wall of your clinic if you perform muscle testing. Not only can it serve as a reminder for possible protocols, it also lets you show your clients what you are checking for. This chart is designed to help you retain clients who may have questions about muscle testing. It is approximately 24 inches long and 18 inches wide.

PRODUCT | Selection Guide

The first product listed below each category on the following pages is often the first choice. Others on the list should also be considered, but they are simply listed in alphabetical order.

- Adrenal Health & Support
- Alkalizing
- Anti-inflammatory
- Antioxidants
- Anxiety
- Athletic Performance & Focus
- Autoimmune
- Betain HCL
- Biotin
- Bladder Health
- Blood Health
- Blood Sugar Support
- Bone Health
- Bowel Health & Function
- Brain Health
- Breast Health
- Bronchial Health
- Calcium Supplementation
- Calming
- Capillary Support
- Cardiovascular Support
- Cellular Health & Support
- Chewable
- Catalyst Complex
- Cholesterol Metabolism
- Choline Supplementation
- Chromium GTF Supplementation
- Circulatory System Support
- Cleansing
- Collagen Support
- Colon Health
- Copper Supplementation
- Cytotrophins
- Dairy Free
- Dental Health, Gums
- Dental Health, Teeth
- Detoxification, Blood
- Detoxification, Cell
- Detoxification, Colon
- Detoxification, Free Radicals & Metal
- Detoxification, Kidney
- Detoxification, Liver
- Digestion, Biliary System
- Digestion, Elimination
- GB Support
- Digestion, Flora
- Digestion, pH
- Digestion, Upper Gastrointestinal Support

- Ear Health
- Emotional Well-Being
- Endocrine Support
- Energy
- Enzomorphogens (EMG)
- Enzymes
- Essential Fatty Acids
- Eye Health
- Fat Metabolism
- Female Hormonal Health
- Fertility Support, Female
- Fertility Support, Male
- Fiber
- Fibrinolytic
- Flexibility
- Folate Supplementation
- Gall Bladder Support
- GastroIntestinal System Support
- Glandulars
- Gluten Free
- Heart Support
- Hemorrhoids
- Homocysteine Management
- Hypothalamus Support
- Immune Support, Acute
- Immune Support, Chronic
- Immune Support, General
- Inflammation
- Inositol Supplementation
- Intestinal Health
- Iodine Support
- Iron Supplementation
- Iron-Free, Multi
- Joint Health & Lubrication Support
- Kidney Health
- Ligament/Tendon Support
- Lipotropic Agent
- Liver Health
- Lung Health
- Lymphatic Function

- Male Hormonal Health
- Magnesium Supplementation
- Manganese Supplementation
- Meal Replacement
- Metabolism Support
- Minerals
- Molybdenum Supplementation
- Multivitamin Support
- Musculoskeletal Function, Acute
- Musculoskeletal Function, Chronic
- Nattokinase
- Nerve Function
- Not Recommended for Pregancy
- Octacosanol
- Omega, Essential Fatty Acids
- Oral Moisture
- Oxygen Metabolism
- Ovary Health
- Pancreas Health
- Parathyroid Health
- Parotid Health
- pH Balance
- Phosphorus Supplementation
- Pineal Health
- Pituitary Health
- Placenta Health
- Potassium Supplementation
- Prebiotic
- Pregnancy Considerations
- Prenatal Support
- Prenatal Support, Final Month
- Probiotic

- Prostate Support
- Protein Shake
- Relaxation
- Respiratory Function
- Selenium Supplementation
- Sinus Support
- Skin and Hair Health
- Sleep Support
- Sneezing & Irritations
- Spinal Support
- Spleen Health
- Sports Health
- Stomach Support
- Stress Support
- Sugar/Sweet Cravings
- Testicular Health
- Thymus Health
- Thyroid Health
- Urinary System Support
- Uterus Health
- Vanadium Supplementation
- Vegetarian Supplementation
- Vitamin A, Alpha & Betacarotene
- Vitamin B Family Supplementation
- Vitamin C Supplementation
- Vitamin D Supplementation
- Vitamin E Supplementation
- Vitamin K Supplementation
- Water Balance
- Weight Management Support
- Zinc Supplementation

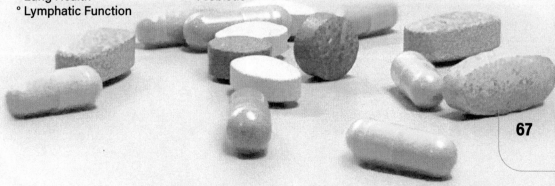

A

Adrenal Health & Support

√ **High Stress Adrenal**
√ **Simply Adrenal**
√ **Vegetarian Adrenal**
» Metabolic Thyro
» Migratrol
» Ligament Complex
» Nerve Chex B
» Vegetarian Tyrosine

Alkalizing

√ **Green Vegetable Alkalizer**
» Land and Sea Minerals

Anti-inflammatory

√ **Inflam-Enzymes**
√ **Herbal Antioxidant**
√ **Turmeric-Boswellia C**
» Advanced Joint Complex
» Omega 3/EPA/DHA

Antioxidants

√ **Herbal Antioxidant**
» Aller-Lung Support
» C Complex
» Cholester-Right
» Complete Ear Health
» Complete Eye Health
» CoQ10-Cardio
» Green Vegetable Alkalizer
» Libida-Life
» Selenium E
» Turmeric-Boswellia C
» Vitamin-Mineral
» Vitamin & Mineral Shake
» Wheat Germ Oil E
» Zinc Complex

Anxiety

√ **Anxie-Tone**
√ **Lith-Mag-Forte**
» Magnesium Complex
» Nerve Chex B
» Restful Mind Support
» Vegetarian Tryptophan

Athletic Performance & Focus

√ **Cardio-Power**
√ **Simply Cardio**
» Anxie-Tone
» Choline Complex
» Vitamin-Mineral
» Vitamin & Mineral Shake
» Wheat Germ Oil E

Autoimmune

» Aller-Lung Support
» Conga-Immune
» Hypothalamus EMG
» Thymo-Immune
» Thymus EMG
» Thyroid EMG

B

Betain HCL

» Digesti-Pan
» Nerve Chex B
» Calcium Lactate +

Biotin

» Anxie-Tone
» B Stress Complex
» Vitamin-Mineral
» Vitamin & Mineral Shake

Bladder Health

√ **Arginase Bladder**
» Green Vegetable Alkalizer
» Kidney Support

Blood Health

√ **Hematic Formula**
√ **Green Vegetable Alkalizer**
√ **Nattokinase**
» Cholester-Right
» Gluco-Sugar-Balance
» Simply Spleen

Blood Sugar Support

√ **Gluco-Sugar-Balance**
√ **Simply Pancreas**
» B Stress Complex
» Beet-Food Plus
» Simply Liver
» Turmeric-Boswellia C
» Vitamin-Mineral
» Vitamin & Mineral Shake

Bone Health

√ **Cal-Mag Complex**
√ **Calcium Complex**
√ **Calcium Lactate +**
» D Complex
» Dento-Gums
» Parathyroid Plus
» Vitamin-Mineral

Bowel Health & Function

√ **Intestinal Support**
» Digesti-Pan
» GB Support
» Intestinal Support
» Probio-Zyme-YST
» Wheat Germ Oil E

Brain Health

√ **Complete Brain Health**
» Herbal Antioxidant
» Lith-Mag-Forte
» Nerve Chex B
» Omega 3/EPA/DHA
» Wheat Germ Oil E

Breast Health

√ **Simply Mammary**
» Feminine Advantage

Bronchial Health

√ **Aller-Lung Support**
» Inflam-Enzymes
» Intracellular Cough
» Simply Lung
» Thymo-Immune

C

Calcium Supplementation

√ **Calcium Complex**
- » Advanced Joint Complex
- » Cal-Mag Complex
- » Calcium Lactate +
- » Catalyst Complex
- » Dento-Gums
- » Ligament Complex
- » Mineral Transport
- » Parathyroid Plus

Calming

√ **Anxie-Tone**
√ **Lith-Mag-Forte**
- » Hypothalamus EMG
- » Inositol Complex
- » Nerve Chex B
- » Simply Hypothalamus
- » Vegetarian Tryptophan

Capillary Support

- » A-C-P Complex

Cardiovascular Support

√ **Cardio-Power**
√ **CoQ10-Cardio**
√ **Simply Cardio**
- » Herbal Antioxidant
- » Nattokinase
- » Selenium E
- » Vegetarian Thyro
- » Vitamin & Mineral Shake

Cellular Health & Support

- » Biofilm Detox
- » Calcium Lactate +
- » Detox-N-Cleanse
- » Omega 3/EPA/DHA
- » Thymus EMG
- » Thyroid EMG
- » Zinc Complex

Chewable

- » Catalyst Complex
- » Dento-Gums

Cholesterol Metabolism

√ **Cholester-Right**
- » Choline Complex
- » GB Support
- » Inositol Complex
- » Liva-DeTox & Support
- » Magnesium Complex
- » Vitamin & Mineral Shake

Choline Supplementation

√ **Choline Complex**
- » Anxie-Tone
- » B Stress Complex
- » Complete Brain Health
- » Nerve Chex B
- » Vitamin-Mineral
- » Vitamin & Mineral Shake

Chromium GTF Supplementation

√ **Gluco-Sugar-Balance**
- » Land and Sea Minerals
- » Metabolic Thyro
- » Migratrol
- » Vitamin-Mineral
- » Vitamin & Mineral Shake

Circulatory System Support

√ **Cardio Power**
- » CoQ10-Cardio
- » Hematic Formula
- » Kidney Support
- » Metabolic Thyro
- » Nattokinase
- » Simply Cardio
- » Kidney Support
- » Vegetarian Adrenal
- » Vegetarian Thyro

Cleansing

- » Beet-Food Plus
- » Biofilm Detox
- » Detox-N-Cleanse
- » Green Vegetable Alkalizer
- » Liva-Detox & Support

Collagen Support

- » Advanced Joint Complex
- » Herbal Antioxidant
- » Ligament Complex

Colon Health

- » Detox-N-Cleanse
- » Intestinal Support
- » Magnesium Complex
- » Lith-Mag-Forte

Copper Supplementation

- » Vitamin-Mineral
- » Vitamin & Mineral Shake

Cytotrophins

- » A-C-P Complex
- » Advanced Joint Complex
- » Anxie-Tone
- » Arginase Bladder
- » Beet-Food Plus
- » Cardio-Power
- » Catalyst Complex
- » Complete Brain Health
- » Complete Ear Health
- » Complete Eye Health
- » Complete Smell & Taste
- » Conga-Immune
- » Digesti-Pan
- » Feminine Advantage
- » GB Support
- » High Stress Adrenal
- » Hypothalamus EMG
- » Intestinal Support
- » Intracellular Cough
- » Kidney Support
- » Ligament Complex
- » Liva-DeTox & Support
- » Masculine Advantage
- » Metabolic Thyro
- » Migratrol
- » Nerve Chex B
- » Parathyroid Plus
- » Pituitary EMG
- » Restful Mind Support
- » Simply Adrenal
- » Simply Cardio
- » Simply Hypothalamus

- » Simply Liver
- » Simply Lung
- » Simply Mammary
- » Simply Orchic
- » Simply Ovary
- » Simply Pancreas
- » Simply Parotid
- » Simply Spleen
- » Simply Thymus
- » Simply Thyroid
- » Simply Uterus
- » Thymo Immune
- » Thymus EMG
- » Thyroid EMG

D

Dairy Free

- » Simply Adrenal
- » Simply Cardio
- » Simply Hypothalamus
- » Simply Liver
- » Simply Lung
- » Simply Mammary
- » Simply Orchic
- » Simply Ovary
- » Simply Pancreas
- » Simply Parotid
- » Simply Spleen
- » Simply Thymus
- » Simply Thyroid
- » Simply Uterus

Dental Health, Gums

√ **Dento-Gums**
- » C Complex
- » CoQ10-Cardio

Dental Health, Teeth

√ **Dento-Gums**
- » Cal-Mag Complex
- » Vitamin-Mineral

Detoxification, Blood

√ **Detox-N-Cleanse**
- » Cholester-Right
- » Complete Ear

- » Green Vegetable Alkalizer
- » Inflam-Enzymes
- » Liva-DeTox & Support
- » Nattokinase
- » Simply Liver
- » Simply Parotid
- » Simply Spleen

Detoxification, Cell

- » Biofilm Detox
- » Herbal Antioxidant
- » Vitamin & Mineral Shake

Detoxification, Colon

√ **Detox-N-Cleanse**
- » Beet-Food Plus
- » Digesti-Pan
- » GB Support
- » Para-Dysbio-Zyme
- » Probio-Zyme-YST

Detoxification, Free Radicals & Metal

√ **Detox-N-Cleanse**
- » C Complex
- » Herbal Antioxidant
- » Simply Parotid

Detoxification, Kidney

√ **Kidney Support**
- » Arginase Bladder
- » Liva-DeTox & Support

Detoxification, Liver

√ **Liva-DeTox & Support**
√ **Simply Liver**
- » Arginase Bladder
- » Beet-Food Plus

Digestion, Biliary System

√ **GB Support**
- » Beet-Food Plus
- » Choline Complex
- » Liva-DeTox & Support
- » Simply Liver
- » Simply Spleen

Digestion, Elimination

√ **GB Support**
- » Beet-Food Plus
- » Digesti-Pan
- » Intestinal Support
- » Liva-DeTox & Support
- » Magnesium Complex
- » Para-Dysbio-Zyme
- » Probio-Zyme-YST
- » Pro-Enzymes

Digestion, Flora

√ **Probio-Zyme-YST**
- » Pro-Enzymes

Digestion, pH

√ **Probio-Zyme-YST**
- » Digesti-Pan
- » Green Vegetable Alkalizer
- » Land and Sea Minerals

Digestion, Salivary

- » Complete Smell & Taste
- » Simply Parotid

Digestion, Upper Gastrointestinal Support

√ **Digesti-Pan**
- » Land and Sea Minerals
- » Para-Dysbio-Zyme
- » Pro-Enzymes
- » Simply Pancreas

E

Ear Health

√ **Complete Ear Health**
- » Magnesium Complex
- » Vitamin-Mineral

Emotional Well-Being

- » Anxie-Tone
- » Choline Complex
- » Complete Brain Health

- » Feminine Advantage
- » Hypothalamus EMG
- » Inositol Complex
- » Libida-Life
- » Lith-Mag-Forte
- » Restful Mind Support
- » Simply Hypothalamus
- » Simply Uterus
- » Vegetarian Tryptophan
- » Vegetarian Tyrosine

Endocrine Support

√ **Hypothalamus EMG**
√ **Simply Hypothalamus**
- » Feminine Advantage
- » Intracellular Cough
- » Pituitary EMG

Energy

√ **Metabolic Thyro**
√ **Simply Thyroid**
- » B Stress Complex
- » Cardio Power
- » Hematic Formula
- » High Stress Adrenal
- » Migratrol
- » Simply Adrenal
- » Simply Cardio
- » Thyroid EMG
- » Vegetarian Adrenal
- » Vegetarian Thyro
- » Vegetarian Tyrosine
- » Wheat Germ Oil E

Enzomorphogens (EMG)

- » Hypothalamus EMG
- » Pituitary EMG
- » Thymus EMG
- » Thyroid EMG

Enzymes

- » Pro-Enzymes
- » Thymus EMG
- » Thyroid EMG

Essential Fatty Acids

- » Omega 3/EPA/DHA
- » Wheat Germ Oil E

Eye Health

√ **Complete Eye Health**
- » Advanced Joint Complex
- » Herbal Antioxidant
- » Vitamin-Mineral

F

Fat Metabolism

√ **GB Support**
- » Beet-Food Plus
- » Choline Complex
- » Inositol Complex
- » Intestinal Support
- » Liva-DeTox & Support
- » Pro-Enzymes
- » Simply Pancreas

Female Hormonal Health

√ **Feminine Advantage**
- » Libida-Life
- » Pituitary EMG
- » Simply Hypothalamus
- » Simply Mammary
- » Simply Ovary
- » Simply Uterus
- » Vitamin-Mineral
- » Vitamin B-6, B-12 & Folate

Fertility Support, Female

√ **Simply Ovary**
- » Libida-Life
- » Vitamin-Mineral

Fertility Support, Male

√ **Masculine Advantage**
- » Libida-Life
- » Simply Orchic
- » Vitamin-Mineral

Fiber

- » Green Vegetable Alkalizer
- » Probio-Zyme-YST
- » Pro-Enzymes
- » Vira-Bac-YST
- » Vitamin & Mineral Shake

Fibrinolytic

√ **Nattokinase**
- » Thymus EMG
- » Thyroid EMG

Flexibility

- » Advanced Joint Complex
- » Inflam-Enzymes
- » Ligament Complex
- » Magnesium Complex

Folate Supplementation

√ **B Stress Complex**
- » Cardio-Power
- » Complete Brain Health
- » Hematic Formula
- » High Stress Adrenal
- » Vegetarian Adrenal
- » Vegetarian Thyro
- » Vitamin-Mineral
- » Vitamin & Mineral Shake
- » Vitamin B-6, B-12 & Folate
- » Vitamin & Mineral Shake

G

Gall Bladder Support

√ **GB Support**
- » Beet-Food Plus
- » Digesti-Pan

GastroIntestinal System Support

√ **GB Support**
√ **Intestinal Support**
- » Digesti-Pan
- » Para-Dysbio-Zyme
- » Probio-Zyme-YST
- » Pro-Enzymes
- » Siimply Pancreas

Glandulars

- » A-C-P Complex
- » Advanced Joint Complex
- » Anxie-Tone
- » Arginase Bladder

- » Beet-Food Plus
- » Cardio-Power
- » Catalyst Complex
- » Complete Brain Health
- » Complete Ear Health
- » Complete Eye Health
- » Complete Smell & Taste
- » Conga-Immune
- » Digesti-Pan
- » Feminine Advantage
- » GB Support
- » High Stress Adrenal
- » Hypothalamus EMG
- » Intestinal Support
- » Intracellular Cough
- » Kidney Support
- » Ligament Complex
- » Liva-DeTox & Support
- » Masculine Advantage
- » Metabolic Thyro
- » Migratrol
- » Nerve Chex B
- » Parathyroid Plus
- » Pituitary EMG
- » Restful Mind Support
- » Simply Adrenal
- » Simply Cardio
- » Simply Hypothalamus
- » Simply Liver
- » Simply Lung
- » Simply Mammary
- » Simply Orchic
- » Simply Ovary
- » Simply Pancreas
- » Simply Parotid
- » Simply Spleen
- » Simply Thymus
- » Simply Thyroid
- » Simply Uterus
- » Thymo Immune
- » Thymus EMG
- » Thyroid EMG
- • *All other glandular-containing Products.*

Gluten Free

- » Advanced Joint Complex
- » Aller-Lung Support
- » Anxie-Tone
- » Arginase Bladder

- » B Stress Complex
- » Biofilm Detox
- » C Complex
- » Calcium Complex
- » Cal-Mag Complex
- » Cardio-Power
- » Cholester-Right
- » Choline Complex
- » Complete Brain Health
- » Complete Ear Health
- » Complete Eye Health
- » Complete Smell & Taste
- » Conga-Immune
- » CoQ10-Cardio
- » D Complex
- » Detox-N-Cleanse
- » Digesti-Pan
- » Feminine Advantage
- » GB Support
- » Gluco-Sugar-Balance
- » Hematic Formula
- » Herbal Antioxidant
- » High Stress Adrenal
- » Hypothalamus EMG
- » Inflam-Enzymes
- » Inositol Complex
- » Intestinal Support
- » Intracellular Cough
- » Kidney Support
- » Land and Sea Minerals
- » Libida-Life
- » Liva-DeTox & Support
- » Magnesium Complex
- » Masculine Advantage
- » Metabolic Thyro
- » Migratrol
- » MIneral Transport
- » Nattokinase
- » Omega 3/EPA/DHA
- » Para-Dysbio-Zyme
- » Pituitary EMG
- » Pro-Enzymes
- » Restful Mind Support
- » Selenium E
- » Simply Adrenal
- » Simply Cardio
- » Simply Hypothalamus
- » Simply Liver
- » Simply Lung
- » Simply Mammary
- » Simply Orchic

- » Simply Ovary
- » Simply Pancreas
- » Simply Parotid
- » Simply Spleen
- » Simply Thymus
- » Simply Thyroid
- » Simply Uterus
- » Thymo Immune
- » Thymus EMG
- » Thyroid EMG
- » Turmeric-Boswellia C
- » Vegetarian Adrenal
- » Vegetarian Thyro
- » Vegetarian Tryptophan
- » Vegetarian Tyrosine
- » Vira-Bac-YST
- » Vira-Chron
- » Vitamin-Mineral
- » Vitamin B-6, B-12 & Folate
- » Zinc Complex

H

Heart Support

√ **Cardio-Power**
√ **CoQ10-Cardio**
√ **Simply Cardio**
- » Intracellular Cough
- » Ligament Complex
- » Nattokinase

Hemorrhoids

- » Intestinal Support

Homocysteine Management

√ **Vitamin B-6, B-12 & Folate**
- » B Stress Complex
- » GB Support

Hypothalamus Support

√ **Simply Hypothalamus**
√ **Hypothalamus EMG**
- » Anxie-Tone
- » High Stress Adrenal
- » Intracellular Cough
- » Nerve Chex B
- » Restful Mind Support

I

Immune Support, Acute

√ **Thymo-Immune**
- » Aller-Lung Support
- » Arginase Bladder
- » C Complex
- » Conga-Immune
- » Herbal Antioxidant
- » Intracellular Cough
- » Simply Thymus
- » Thymus EMG
- » Vira-Bac-YST
- » Vira-Chron
- » Zinc Complex

Immune Support, Chronic

√ **Thymo-Immune**
- » Aller-Lung Support
- » Catalyst Complex
- » Conga-Immune
- » Intracellular Cough
- » Simply Spleen
- » Vira-Bac-YST
- » Vira-Chron
- » Vitamin-Mineral
- » Zinc Complex

Immune Support, General

- » Aller-Lung Support
- » Arginase Bladder
- » Catalyst Complex
- » Conga-Immune
- » D Complex
- » Intracellular Cough
- » Vitamin-Mineral
- » Vitamin & Mineral Shake
- » Wheat Germ Oil E

Inflammation

√ **Inflam-Enzymes**
- » Advanced Joint Complex
- » Herbal Antioxidant
- » Omega 3/EPA/DHA
- » Turmeric-Boswellia C

Inositol Supplementation

√ **Inositol Complex**
- » Anxie-Tone
- » B Stress Complex
- » Complete Brain Health
- » High Stress Adrenal
- » Ligament Complex
- » Vitamin-Mineral

Intestinal Health

√ **Intestinal Support**
- » Digesti-Pan
- » GB Support
- » Para-Dysbio-Zyme
- » Probio-Zyme-YST
- » Pro-Enzymes

Iron Supplementation

√ **Hematic Formula**
- » Vitamin-Mineral

Iron-Free, Multi

- » Catalyst Complex
- » Vitamin & Mineral Shake

J

Joint Health & Lubrication Support

√ **Advanced Joint Complex**
- » Cal-Mag Complex
- » Inflam-Enzymes
- » Ligament Complex
- » Magnesium Complex
- » Omega 3/EPA/DHA
- » Turmeric-Boswellia C

K

Kidney Health

√ **Kidney Support**
- » A-C-P Complex
- » Arginase Bladder
- » Green Vegetable Alkalizer

L

Ligament/Tendon Support

√ **Ligament Complex**
√ **Advanced Joint Complex**
- » Cal-Mag Complex
- » Inflam-Enzymes
- » Magnesium Complex

Lipotropic Agent

√ **Beet-Food Plus**
- » Cholester-Right
- » Choline Complex
- » Digesti-Pan
- » GB Support
- » Inositol Complex

Liver Health

√ **Liva-DeTox & Support**
√ **Simply Liver**
- » Beet-Food Plus
- » Choline Complex
- » GB Support
- » Green Vegetable Alkalizer
- » Inositol Complex
- » Intestinal Support
- » Intracellular Cough
- » Kidney Support
- » Vira-Chron

Lung Health

√ **Simply Lung**
- » Aller-Lung Support
- » Inflam-Enzymes
- » Intracellular Cough
- » Land and Sea Minerals

Lymphatic Function

√ **Simply Spleen**
- » A-C-P Complex
- » Aller-Lung Support
- » Intestinal Support
- » Intracellular Cough
- » Liva-DeTox & Support
- » Simply Liver
- » Simply Thymus
- » Thymo-Immune
- » Thymus EMG

M

Male Hormonal Health

√ Masculine Advantage
- » Libida-Life
- » Simply Orchic
- » Vitamin-Mineral

Magnesium Supplementation

√ Magnesium Complex
- » Advanced Joint Complex
- » Cal-Mag Complex
- » Calcium Lactate +
- » Catalyst Complex
- » Inflam-Enzymes
- » Lith-Mag-Forte
- » Mineral Transport
- » Nerve Chex B
- » Parathyroid Plus

Manganese Supplementation

√ Inflam-Enzymes
- » Cal-Mag Complex
- » Nerve Chex B
- » Vitamin-Mineral
- » Vitamin & Mineral Shake

Meal Replacement

- » Vitamin & Mineral Shake

Metabolism Support

√ Metabolic Thyro
- » Migratrol
- » Pituitary EMG
- » Simply Hypothalamus
- » Simply Liver
- » Simply Pancreas
- » Simply Thyroid
- » Thyroid EMG
- » Vegetarian Thyro

Minerals

√ Land and Sea Minerals
- » Calcium Lactate +

- » Ligament Complex
- » Magnesium Complex
- » Nerve Chex B
- » Vitamin-Mineral
- » Vitamin & Mineral Shake

Molybdenum Supplementation

- » Vitamin-Mineral
- » Vitamin & Mineral Shake

Mood Support

√ Anxie-Tone
√ Complete Brain Health
- » Choline Complex
- » Feminine Advantage
- » High Stress Adrenal
- » Hypothalamus EMG
- » Inositol Complex
- » Land and Sea Minerals
- » Libida-Life
- » Lith-Mag-Forte
- » Magnesium Complex
- » Masculine Advantage
- » Metabolic Thyro
- » Migratrol
- » Mineral Transport
- » Nerve Chex B
- » Omega 3/EPA/DHA
- » Pituitary EMG
- » Restful Mind Support
- » Simply Hypothalamus
- » Simply Orchic
- » Simply Ovary
- » Simply Thyroid
- » Simply Uterus
- » Thyroid EMG
- » Vegetarian Thyro
- » Vegetarian Tryptophan
- » Vegetarian Tyrosine
- » Wheat Germ Oil E

Multivitamin Support

√ Vitamin-Mineral
- » Catalyst Complex
- » Vitamin & Mineral Shake

Musculoskeletal Function, Acute

√ Inflam-Enzymes
- » Advanced Joint Complex
- » Cardio-Power
- » Magnesium Complex
- » Omega 3/EPA/DHA

Musculoskeletal Function, Chronic

√ Cal-Mag Complex
- » Advanced Joint Complex
- » Calcium Lactate +
- » Cardio-Power
- » D Complex
- » Ligament Complex
- » Omega 3/EPA/DHA
- » Simply Cardio

N

Nattokinase

- » Nattokinase

Nerve Function

√ Anxie-Tone
- » B Stress Complex
- » Calcium Lactate +
- » Choline Complex
- » Complete Brain Health
- » Hypothalamus EMG
- » Inositol Complex
- » Libida-Life
- » Lith-Mag-Forte
- » Nerve Chex B
- » Omega 3/EPA/DHA
- » Restful Mind Support
- » Simply Hypothalamus
- » Vegetarian Tryptophan
- » Vegetarian Tyrosine
- » Vitamin B6, B12, & Folate
- » Wheat Germ Oil E

Not Recommended for Pregancy

- » Migratrol

» Para-Dysbio-Zyme
» Thymo-Immune
» Vegetarian Thyro

O

Octacosanol

» Wheat Germ Oil E

Omega, Essential Fatty Acids

√ Omega 3/EPA/DHA
» Wheat Germ Oil E

Oral Moisture

» Complete Smell & Taste
» Simply Parotid

Oxygen Metabolism

√ Cardio-Power
» C Complex
» CoQ10-Cardio
» Hematic Formula
» Herbal Antioxidant
» Selenium E
» Wheat Germ Oil E

Ovary Health

√ Simply Ovary
» Feminine Advantage

P

Pancreas Health

√ Simply Pancreas
» Digesti-Pan
» Gluco-Sugar-Balance
» Intestinal Support
» Kidney Support
» Vitamin-Mineral

Parathyroid Health

√ Parathyroid Plus
» Cal-Mag Complex
» Intracellular Cough

Parotid Health

√ Simply Parotid
» Complete Smell & Taste
» Restful Mind Support

pH Balance

√ Acidifiers
» Arginase Bladder
» Digesti-Pan
√ Alkalizers
» Green Vegetable Alkalizer
√ Normalizers
» Land and Sea Minerals
» Probio-Zyme-YST

Phosphorus Supplementation

» D Complex
» Vitamin & Mineral Shake
▪ *All food products naturally contain phosphorus.*

Pineal Health

√ Restful Mind Support
» Intracellular Cough
» Vegetarian Tryptophan

Pituitary Health

√ Pituitary EMG
» Hypothalamus EMG
» Intracellular Cough
» Metabolic Thyro
» Migratrol
» Restful Mind Support
» Simply Hypothalamus
» Vegetarian Thyro

Placenta Health

» Simply Uterus

Potassium Supplementation

√ Green Vegetable Alkalizer
» Land and Sea Minerals
» Vitamin & Mineral Shake
▪ *All food products naturally*

contain potassium, excluding oils.

Prebiotic

» Probio-Zyme-YST

Pregnancy Considerations

√ Vitamin-Mineral
» Hypothalamus EMG
» Pituitary EMG
» Simply Adrenal
» Simply Cardio
» Simply Hypothalamus
» Simply Liver
» Simply Lung
» Simply Mammary
» Simply Orchic
» Simply Ovary
» Simply Pancreas
» Simply Parotid
» Simply Spleen
» Simply Thymus
» Simply Thyroid
» Thymus EMG
» Thyroid EMG
» Vitamin-Mineral

Prenatal Support

√ Vitamin-Mineral
» Calcium Complex
» Hematic Formula
» Magnesium Complex

Prenatal Support, Final Month

√ Simply Uterus
√ Vitamin-Mineral
» Calcium Complex
» Magnesium Complex

Probiotic

» Probio-Zyme-YST

Prostate Support

» Masculine Advantage
» Simply Orchic

Protein Shake

- » Vitamin & Mineral Shake

R

Relaxation

- » Anxie-Tone
- » Complete Brain Health
- » Lith-Mag-Forte
- » Restful Mind Support
- » Simply Adrenal

Respiratory Function

√ **Aller-Lung Support**
√ **Simply Lung**
- » Inflam-Enzymes
- » Intracellular Cough
- » Thymo-Immune
- » Vira-Bac-YST

S

Selenium Supplementation

√ **Selenium E**
- » Cardio-Power
- » Complete Brain Health
- » Complete Eye Health
- » Herbal Antioxidant
- » Masculine Advantage
- » Vitamin-Mineral
- » Vitamin & Mineral Shake

Sinus Support

√ **Aller-Lung Support**
- » C Complex
- » Simply Lung
- » Vira-Chron

Skin and Hair Health

√ **Vitamin-Mineral**
- » Advanced Joint Complex
- » Green Vegetable Alkalizer
- » Herbal Antioxidant
- » Omega 3/EPA/DHA

- » Simply Thymus
- » Thymo-Immune
- » Thymus EMG
- » Vitamin-Mineral
- » Vitamin & Mineral Shake
- » Wheat Germ Oil E
- » Zinc Complex

Sleep Support

√ **Restful Mind Support**
- » Calcium Complex
- » Feminine Advantage
- » Magnesium Complex
- » Pituitary EMG
- » Simply Hypothalamus
- » Simply Ovary
- » Vegetarian Tryptophan

Sneezing & Irritants

√ **Aller-Lung Support**
- » C Complex
- » Herbal Antioxidant

Spinal Support

√ **Inflam-Enzymes**
- » Advanced Joint Complex
- » Cal-Mag Complex
- » Calcium Lactate +
- » Dento-Gums
- » Ligament Complex
- » Magnesium Complex
- » Omega 3/EPA/DHA

Spleen Health

√ **Simply Spleen**
- » GB Support

Sports Health

√ **Cardio-Power**
- » Advanced Joint Complex
- » Choline Complex
- » Metabolic Thyro
- » Simply Adrenal
- » Simply Cardio
- » Vitamin-Mineral
- » Vitamin & Mineral Shake
- » Wheat Germ Oil E

Stress Support

- » Anxie-Tone
- » B Stress Complex
- » High Stress Adrenal
- » Inositiol Complex
- » Lith-Mag-Forte
- » Magnesium Complex
- » Metabolic Thyro
- » Migratrol
- » Nerve Chex B
- » Restful Mind Support
- » Simply Adrenal
- » Simply Orchic
- » Siimply Uterus
- » Vegetarian Adrenal
- » Vegetarian Thyro
- » Vegetarian Tryptophan
- » Vegetarian Tyrosine

Sugar/Sweet Cravings

√ **Gluco-Sugar-Balance**
- » Beet-Food Plus
- » Land and Sea Minerals
- » Turmeric-Boswellia C
- » Vitamin-Mineral
- » Vitamin & Mineral Shake

T

Testicular Health

√ **Simply Orchic**
- » Libida Life
- » Masculine Advantage
- » Simply Parotid
- » Zinc Complex

Thymus Health

√ **Simply Thymus**
√ **Thymo-Immune**
√ **Thymus EMG**
- » Conga-Immune
- » Intracellular Cough

Thyroid Health

√ **Simply Thyroid**
√ **Thyroid EMG**
√ **Metabolic Thyro**

- » Green Vegetable Alkalizer
- » Intracellular Cough
- » Migratrol
- » Mineral Transport
- » Pituitary EMG
- » Selenium E
- » Simply Hypothalamus
- » Simply Parotid
- » Vegetarian Thyro
- » Vegetarian Tyrosine
- » Vitamin-Mineral

U

Urinary System Support

- » Arginase Bladder
- » Kidney Support

Urination, Excessive

- » Arginase Bladder
- » Masculine Advantage

Urination, Irritation

- » Thymo-Immune
- » Vira-Bac-YST

Uterus Health

- √ **Simply Uterus**
- » Libida-Life
- » Feminine Advantage

V

Vanadium Supplementation

- » Gluco-Sugar-Balance
- » Vitamin-Mineral

Vegetarian Supplementation

- » Aller-Lung Support
- » B Stress Complex
- » Beet-Food Plus
- » Biofilm Detox
- » C Complex
- » Calcium Complex

- » Cal-Mag Complex
- » Calcium Complex
- » Cholester-Right
- » Choline Complex
- » CoQ10-Cardio
- » D Complex
- » Detox-N-Cleanse
- » Gluco-Sugar-Balance
- » Green Vegetable Alkalizer
- » Hematic Formula
- » Herbal Antioxidant
- » Inflam-Enzymes
- » Inositol Complex
- » Land and Sea Minerals
- » Libida-Life
- » Magnesium Complex
- » Mineral Transport
- » Nattokinase
- » Para-Dysbio-Zyme
- » Pro-Enzymes
- » Probio-Zyme-YST
- » Selenium E
- » Turmeric-Boswellia C
- » Vegetarian Adrenal
- » Vegetarian Thyro
- » Vegetarian Tryptophan
- » Vegetarian Tyrosine
- » Vira-Bac-YST
- » Vira-Chron
- » Vitamin-Mineral
- » Vitamin & Mineral Shake
- » Vitamin B6, B12, & Folate
- » Zinc Complex

Vitamin A, Alpha & Betacarotene

- √ **Vitamin-Mineral**
- √ **Vitamin & Mineral Shake**
- » A-C-P Complex
- » Beet-Food Plus
- » Catalyst Complex
- » Complete Eye Health
- » Herbal Antioxidant
- » Ligament Complex

Vitamin B Family Supplementation

- √ **B Stress Complex**
- √ **Nerve Chex B**
- √ **Vitamin B6, B12, & Folate**

- » Anxie-Tone
- » Beet-Food Plus
- » Cardio-Power
- » Catalyst Complex
- » Complete Brain Health
- » Hematic Formula
- » High Stress Adrenal
- » Ligament Complex
- » Vitamin-Mineral
- » Vitamin & Mineral Shake
- » Vitamin B6, B12, & Folate

Vitamin C Supplementation

- √ **C Complex**
- √ **A-C-P Complex**
- √ **Turmeric-Boswellia C**
- » Advanced Joint Complex
- » Aller-Lung Support
- » Anxie-Tone
- » Arginase Bladder
- » Cal-Mag Complex
- » Cardio-Power
- » Catalyst Complex
- » Cholester-Right
- » Complete Brain Health
- » Complete Ear Health
- » Complete Eye Health
- » Conga-Immune
- » CoQ10-Cardio
- » Dento-Gums
- » Detox-N-Cleanse
- » Hematic Formula
- » Herbal Antioxidant
- » High Stress Adrenal
- » Inflam-Enzymes
- » Intracellular Cough
- » Kidney Support
- » Ligament Complex
- » Nerve Chex B
- » Thymo-Immune
- » Vegetarian Adrenal
- » Vitamin-Mineral
- » Vitamin & Mineral Shake

Vitamin D Supplementation

- √ **D Complex**
- » Advanced Joint Complex
- » Cal-Mag Complex

- » Catalyst Complex
- » Ligament Complex
- » Parathyroid Plus
- » Vitamin-Mineral
- » Vitamin & Mineral Shake

Vitamin E Supplementation

√ **Selenium E**
√ **Wheat Germ Oil E**
- » A-C-P Complex
- » Beet-Food Plus
- » Cardio-Power
- » Complete Brain Health
- » Complete Eye Health
- » Herbal Antioxidant
- » Ligament Complex
- » Masculine Advantage
- » Omega 3/EPA/DHA
- » Vitamin-Mineral
- » Vitamin & Mineral Shake

Vitamin K Supplementation

- » Cal-Mag Complex
- » Green Vegetable Alkalizer
- » Vitamin-Mineral
- » Vitamin & Mineral Shake

W

Water Balance

- » Arginase Bladder
- » Green Vegetable Alkalizer
- » Kidney Support
- » Simply Hypothalamus

Weight Management Support

√ **All thyroid support supplement**
- » Gluco-Sugar-Balance
- » Green Vegetable Alkalizer

- » Vitamin-Mineral
- » Vitamin & Mineral Shake

Z

Zinc Supplementation

√ **Zinc Complex**
- » Advanced Joint Complex
- » Complete Ear Health
- » Complete Eye Health
- » Complete Smell & Taste
- » Conga-Immune
- » Herbal Antioxidant
- » High Stress Adrenal
- » Libida-Life
- » Probio-Zyme-YST
- » Vegatarian Thyro
- » Vitamin-Mineral
- » Vitamin & Mineral Shake

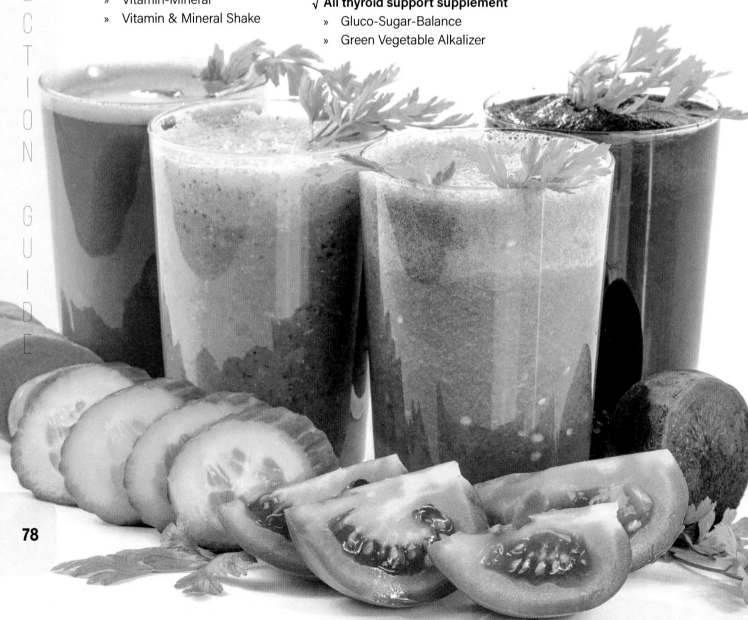

PRODUCT | INGREDIENTS/COMPONENTS CROSS REFERENCE

The ingredients and components in this list are often in multiple products. The products are simply listed in alphabetical order. Not all products are listed (mainly if the amount was quite low). A component is something that is naturally present in the food, but not necessarily added as a separate ingredient—nor is its presence necessarily tested for.

For example, while products with bovine tracheal cartilage naturally contain chondroitin sulfate and glucosamine sulfate, those items are not extracted out of it in our products.

A

Acerola Cherry

- » A-C-P Complex
- » Advanced Joint Complex
- » Aller-Lung Support
- » Anxie-Tone
- » Arginase Bladder
- » C Complex
- » Cardio-Power
- » Catalyst Complex
- » Cholester Right
- » Complete Brain Health
- » Complete Ear Health
- » Complete Eye Health
- » Conga-Immune
- » CoQ10-Cardio
- » Dento-Gums
- » Detox-N-Cleanse
- » Herbal Antioxidant
- » High Stress Adrenal
- » Inflam-Enzymes
- » Intracellular Cough
- » Kidney Support
- » Ligament Complex
- » Nerve Chex B
- » Thymo-Immune
- » Turmeric-Boswellia C
- » Vegetarian Adrenal
- » Vitamin-Mineral
- » Vitamin & Mineral Shake

Acidophilus, Non-dairy

- » Pro-Enzymes
- » Probio-Zyme-YST
- » Vitamin & Mineral Shake

Adrenal, Bovine

√ **High Stress Adrenal**
√ **Simply Adrenal**
(an alternative could be Vegetarian Adrenal)
- » A-C-P Complex
- » Catalyst Complex
- » Dento-Gums
- » Ligament Complex
- » Metabolic Thyro
- » Migratrol

African Pygeum

- » Masculine Advantage

Alfalfa

- » A-C-P Complex
- » Advanced Joint Complex
- » Anxie-Tone
- » Beet-Food Plus
- » Catalyst Complex
- » Conga-Immune
- » Green Vegetable Alkalizer
- » Land and Sea Minerals
- » Metabolic Thyro
- » Mineral Transport
- » Vitamin-Mineral
- » Vitamin & Mineral Shake

Almonds

- » Para-Dysbio-Zyme

Aloe Vera

- » Advanced Joint Complex

Alpha-Linolenic Acid

- » Complete Brain Health *(in flax)*

Alpha Lipoic Acid

- » Complete Brain Health

Amygdalin

- » Para-Dysbio-Zyme

Amylase

- » Digesti-Pan
- » Green Vegetable Alkalizer
- » Pro-Enzymes
- » Simply Pancreas
- » Vitamin & Mineral Shake

Angelica

- » Vira-Chron

Apple Pectin *(Fiber)*

- » Cholester-Right
- » Detox-N-Cleanse

Arginase, Bovine

√ **Arginase Bladder**
- » Liva-DeTox & Support
- » Simply Liver

Artichoke Leaf

- » Probio-Zyme-YST

Ashwagandha

- » Vegetarian Adrenal

Astragalus

- » Biofilm Detox
- » Inflam-Enzymes
- » Libida-Life
- » Para-Dysbio-Zyme
- » Thymo-Immune

B

Barley Grass

- » Green Vegetable Alkalizer
- » Vitamin & Mineral Shake

Beet Root/Leaf

- √ **Beet-Food Plus**
- » Arginase Bladder
- » Digesti-Pan
- » GB Support
- » Hematic Formula
- » Kidney Support
- » Ligament Complex
- » Liva-DeTox & Support
- » Nattokinase
- » Pro-Enzymes
- » Probio-Zyme-YST
- » Vira-Bac-YST
- » Vitamin B6, B12, & Folate

Benfotiamine *(in Garlic)*

- » Cardio-Power
- » Kidney Support
- » Liva-DeTox & Support
- » Para-Dysbio-Zyme
- » Thymo-Immune

Berberine

- » Gluco-Sugar-Balance

Betacarotene *(Vitamin A)*

- √ **Complete Eye Health**
- » A-C-P Complex
- » Beet-Food Plus
- » Complete Eye Health
- » Catalyst Complex
- » Herbal Antioxidant
- » Ligament Complex

- » Vitamin-Mineral
- » Vitamin & Mineral Shake

Beta-Glucans

- » Cholester-Right

Beta-Glucanase

- » Biofilm Detox

Betaine HCL

- √ **Digesti-Pan**
- » Calcium Lactate +
- » Nerve Chex B

Beta-Sitosterol

- » Masculine Advantage *(in Saw Palmetto)*

Bilberry Berries

- » Biofilm Detox
- » Complete Eye Health

Bile, Bovine Ox

- » GB Support
- » Intestinal Support

Bioflavonoids

- » A-C-P Complex
- » Advanced Joint Complex
- » Aller-Lung Support
- » Anxie-Tone
- » Arginase Bladder
- » Cardio-Power
- » Catalyst Complex
- » Cholester-Right
- » Complete Brain Health
- » Complete Ear Health
- » Complete Eye Health
- » Conga-Immune
- » CoQ10-Cardio
- » Dento-Gums
- » Detox-N-Cleanse
- » Herbal Antioxidant
- » High Stress Adrenal
- » Inflam-Enzymes
- » Intracellular Cough
- » Kidney Support

- » Ligament Complex
- » Nerve Chex B
- » Thymo-Immune
- » Turmeric-Boswellia C
- » Vegetarian Adrenal

Biogurt *(Lactobacillus Bulgaricus)*

- » Catalyst Complex
- » Magnesium Complex
- » Mineral Transport
- » Parathyroid Plus

Biotin, Food *(Vitamin B-7)*

- √ **B Stress Complex**
- » Anxie-Tone
- » Vitamin-Mineral
- » Vitamin & Mineral Shake

Bitter Citrus

- » Aller-Lung Support

Bitter Melon

- » Gluco-Sugar-Balance

Black Cohosh

- » Feminine Advantage

Black Walnut

- √ **Para-Dysbio-Zyme**
- » Biofilm Detox

Bladderwrack

- » Arginase Bladder

Bone Marrow, Bovine

- » A-C-P Complex
- » Conga-Immune
- » Dento-Gums
- » Ligament Complex

Bone Meal, Bovine

- » A-C-P Complex
- » Catalyst Complex
- » Dento-Gums
- » Ligament Complex

Boron, Food

- » Advanced Joint Complex
- » Cal-Mag Complex
- » Vitamin-Mineral
- » Vitamin & Mineral Shake

Boswellia Gum

- » Turmeric-Boswellia C

Brain, Bovine

- √ **Complete Brain Health**
- » Nerve Chex B

Broccoli

- » Complete Eye Health
- » Metabolic Thyro

Bromelain

- » Aller-Lung Support
- » Inflam-Enzymes
- » Intracellular Cough
- » Para-Dysbio-Zyme

Bromine, Food *(in Kelp)*

- » Metabolic Thyro
- » Vegetarian Thyro

Brown Rice

- » A-C-P Complex
- » Aller-Lung Support
- » Anxie-Tone
- » Arginase Bladder
- » B Stress Complex
- » Cardio-Power
- » Catalyst Complex
- » Cholester-Right
- » Complete Brain Health
- » Complete Eye Health
- » Conga-Immune
- » CoQ10-Cardio
- » Dento-Gums
- » GB Support
- » High Stress Adrenal
- » Intracellular Cough
- » Ligament Complex
- » Masculine Advantage
- » Selenium E

- » Simply Adrenal
- » Simply Cardio
- » Simply Liver
- » Simply Orchic
- » Simply Ovary
- » Simply Parotid
- » Thymus EMG
- » Thyroid EMG
- » Vegetarian Adrenal
- » Vitamin-Mineral
- » Vitamin & Mineral Shake

Buckwheat

- » A-C-P Complex
- » Arginase Bladder
- » Conga-Immune
- » Kidney Support
- » Vira-Bac-YST

Bupleurum

- » Vira-Chron

Burdock

- » Advanced Joint Complex
- » Metabolic Thyro
- » Para-Dysbio-Zyme
- » Vegetarian Thyro

C

Cabbage

- » Probio-Zyme-YST

Calcium, Food

- √ **Calcium Complex**
- » Advanced Joint Complex
- » Beet-Food Plus
- » Cal-Mag Complex
- » Calcium Lactate +
- » Catalyst Complex
- » Dento-Gums
- » Inflam-Enzymes
- » Ligament Complex
- » Mineral Transport
- » Nerve Chex B
- » Parathyroid Plus

Caprylic Acid

- » Probio-Zyme-YST

Carbamide

- » Ligament Complex

Cardiac Muscle Cytotrophin

- » Simply Cardio

Carob *(Pod)*

- » Vegetarian Adrenal

Carrots

- » A-C-P Complex
- » Arginase Bladder
- » Beet-Food Plus
- » Catalyst Complex
- » Complete Eye Health
- » Conga-Immune
- » Dento-Gums
- » GB Support
- » Intracellular Cough
- » Kidney Support
- » Ligament Complex
- » Para-Dysbio-Zyme
- » Thymo-Immune
- » Vegetarian Thyro
- » Vitamin-Mineral
- » Vitamin & Mineral Shake

Cartilage, Bovine

- » Advanced Joint Complex
- » Dento-Gums
- » Ligament Complex

Cat's Claw

- » Kidney Support

Cayenne Fruit

- » Advanced Joint Complex
- » Thymo-Immune

Cellulase

- » Biofilm Detox

» Green Vegetable Alkalizer
» Para-Dysbio-Zyme
» Pro-Enzymes
» Probio-Zyme-YST
» Vitamin & Mineral Shake

Celery

» Green Vegetable Alkalizer
» Vitamin & Mineral Shake

Chaga

» Organic Mushrooms

Chaste Tree Berries

» Feminine Advantage

Chinese Thoroughwax

» Complete Ear Health

Chlorella

» Detox-N-Cleanse

Chlorophyll
(in Green Plants)

» Beet-Food Plus
» Cal-Mag Complex
» Calcium Complex
» Catalyst Complex
» Conga-Immune
» Detox-N-Cleanse
» Green Vegetable Alkalizer
» Land and Sea Minerals
» Magnesium Complex
» Metabolic Thyro
» Vira-Bac-YST
» Vitamin-Mineral
» Vitamin & Mineral Shake

Choline

√ **Choline Complex**
» Anxie-Tone
» B Stress Complex
» Complete Brain Health
» High Stress Adrenal
» Nerve Chex B
» Vitamin-Mineral

Chondroitin Sulfate
(in Trachea)

» Advanced Joint Complex
» Complete Brain Health
» Complete Eye Health

Chromium GTF, Food

» Gluco-Sugar-Balance
» Land and Sea Minerals
» Metabolic Thyro
» Migratrol
» Vitamin-Mineral
» Vitamin & Mineral Shake

Chymotrypsin, Bovine

» Hypothalamus EMG
» Pituitary EMG
» Simply Pancreas
» Thymus EMG
» Thyroid EMG

Cilantro

» Detox-N-Cleanse

Cinnamon

» Gluco-Sugar-Balance
» Intestinal Support
» Probio-Zyme-YST
» Vitamin & Mineral Shake

Citrus Aurantium

» Probio-Zyme-YST

Citrus Bioflavonoids

» Aller-Lung Support
» C Complex
» Cal-Mag Complex
» Herbal Antioxidant
» Hematic Formula
» High Stress Adrenal
» Vitamin-Mineral

Citrus Pectin

» Detox-N-Cleanse

Clove

» Para-Dysbio-Zyme
» Probio-Zyme-YST

Coconut Oil

» Probio-Zyme-YST

Cod Liver Oil

» Complete Eye Health

CoEnzyme Q10

√ **CoQ10-Cardio**
» Cardio-Power
» Complete Ear Health
» Simply Cardio

Collagen Peptides

» Ligament Complex

Collinsonia Root

» Anxie-Tone
» Detox-N-Cleanse
» GB Support
» Hypothalamus EMG
» Intestinal Support
» Lith-Mag-Forte
» Pituitary EMG
» Thymus EMG
» Thyroid EMG

Copper, Food

» Vitamin-Mineral
» Vitamin & Mineral Shake

Coptis

» Vira-Chron

Cordyceps

» Catalyst Complex
» Dual Vitality
» Organic Mushrooms

Corn Silk

» Complete Brain Health
» Kidney Support

Cytotrophins

- » A-C-P Complex
- » Advanced Joint Complex
- » Anxie-Tone
- » Arginase Bladder
- » Beet-Food Plus
- » Cardio-Power
- » Catalyst Complex
- » Complete Brain Health
- » Complete Ear Health
- » Complete Eye Health
- » Complete Smell & Taste
- » Conga-Immune
- » Digesti-Pan
- » Feminine Advantage
- » GB Support
- » High Stress Adrenal
- » Hypothalamus EMG
- » Intestinal Support
- » Intracellular Cough
- » Kidney Support
- » Ligament Complex
- » Liva-DeTox & Support
- » Masculine Advantage
- » Metabolic Thyro
- » Migratrol
- » Nerve Chex B
- » Parathyroid Plus
- » Pituitary EMG
- » Restful Mind Support
- » Simply Adrenal
- » Simply Cardio
- » Simply Hypothalamus
- » Simply Liver
- » Simply Lung
- » Simply Mammary
- » Simply Orchic
- » Simply Ovary
- » Simply Pancreas
- » Simply Parotid
- » Simply Spleen
- » Simply Thymus
- » Simply Thyroid
- » Simply Uterus
- » Thymo Immune
- » Thymus EMG
- » Thyroid EMG

D

Damiana

- » Masculine Advantage

Dandelion

- » Kidney Support

Deoxyribonucleic Acid

- » Complete Brain Health

Devil's Claw

- » Advanced Joint Complex

DHEA *(in Bovine Adrenals)*

- » A-C-P Complex
- » Catalyst Complex
- » High Stress Adrenal
- » Ligament Complex
- » Metabolic Thyro
- » Migratrol
- » Simply Adrenal

Diindolylmethane *(in Broccoli)*

- » Complete Eye Health
- » Metabolic Thyro

Dong Quai Root

- » Migratrol
- » Vegetarian Thyro

Docosahexaenoic Acid (DHA)

- » Omega 3/EPA/DHA

E

Ear, Fish

- » Complete Ear Health

Echinacea Purpurea Root

- √ Conga-Immune
- » A-C-P Complex

- » Biofilm Detox
- » Thymo-Immune

Eicosapentaenoic Acid (EPA)

- » Omega 3/EPA/DHA

Elderberry

- » Intracellular Cough

Eleuthero Root *(Siberian Ginseng)*

- » Complete Brain Health
- » Herbal Antioxidant
- » High Stress Adrenal
- » Thymo-Immune

Endopeptidase/ Exopeptidase

- » Biofilm Detox

Endothelium/Epithelium

- » Advanced Joint Complex
- » Complete Brain Health

Enzymes, Digestive

- » Digesti-Pan
- » Green Vegetable Alkalizer
- » Inflam-Enzymes
- » Para-Dysbio-Zyme
- » Probio-Zyme-YST
- » Pro-Enzymes
- » Vitamin & Mineral Shake

Essential Fatty Acids

- √ Omega 3/EPA/DHA
- » Complete Brain Health
- » Complete Eye Health
- » Feminine Advantage
- » Ligament Complex
- » Masculine Advantage
- » Migratrol
- » Wheat Germ Oil E

Eye, Fish

- » Complete Eye Health

Eyebright

- » Complete Eye Health

F

Fenugreek

- » Aller-Lung-Support
- » Gluco-Sugar-Balance
- » Metabolic Thyro
- » Turmeric-Boswellia C

Feverfew Leaves

- » Migratrol

Fiber

- » Green Vegetable Alkalizer
- » Pro-Enzymes
- » Vitamin & Mineral Shake

Figs

- » Para-Dysbio-Zyme

Fish Oil, Herring

- » Omega 3/EPA/DHA

Flaxseeds

√ **Complete Brain Health**
- » Advanced Joint Complex
- » Beet-Food Plus
- » Feminine Advantage
- » Ligament Complex
- » Masculine Advantage
- » Migratrol

Folate, Food (Vitamin B-9)

- » Anxie-Tone
- » B Stress Complex
- » Cardio-Power
- » Complete Brain Health
- » Hematic Formula
- » High Stress Adrenal
- » Vegetarian Adrenal
- » Vegetarian Thyro
- » Vitamin-Mineral
- » Vitamin & Mineral Shake
- » Vitamin B-6, B-12 & Folate

Folic Acid

- ▪ *No FOOD product supplies folic acid as it is not food. Foods supply folate as vitamin B-9 source.*

Forsythia

- » Vira-Chron

French Lilac

- ▪ *See Goat's Rue*

G

Gamma Linolenic Acid

- » Migratrol
- » Wheat Germ Oil E

Gardenia

- » Vira-Chron

Garlic

- » Biofilm Detox
- » Cardio-Power
- » Cholester-Right
- » Conga-Immune
- » CoQ10-Cardio
- » Detox-N-Cleanse
- » Kidney Support
- » Liva-DeTox & Support
- » Para-Dysbio-Zyme
- » Probio-Zyme-YST
- » Thymo-Immune

Gelatin, Bovine (Gelcap)

- » Omega 3/EPA/DHA

Gentian Root

- » Pro-Enzymes

Ginger Rhizome/Root

- » Cholester-Right
- » Digesti-Pan
- » Herbal Antioxidant
- » Pro-Enzymes
- » Turmeric-Boswellia C

Ginkgo Biloba

- » Anxie-Tone
- » Complete Ear Health
- » Complete Eye Health
- » Herbal Antioxidant

Ginseng, American

- » Dual Vitality

Ginseng, Korean Red

- » Masculine Advantage

Ginseng, Siberian

- ▪ *See Eleuthero Root*

Glandulars

- » A-C-P Complex
- » Advanced Joint Complex
- » Anxie-Tone
- » Arginase Bladder
- » Beet-Food Plus
- » Cardio-Power
- » Catalyst Complex
- » Complete Brain Health
- » Complete Ear Health
- » Complete Eye Health
- » Complete Smell & Taste
- » Conga-Immune
- » Digesti-Pan
- » Feminine Advantage
- » GB Support
- » High Stress Adrenal
- » Hypothalamus EMG
- » Intestinal Support
- » Intracellular Cough
- » Kidney Support
- » Ligament Complex
- » Liva-DeTox & Support
- » Masculine Advantage
- » Metabolic Thyro
- » Migratrol
- » Nerve Chex B
- » Parathyroid Plus
- » Pituitary EMG
- » Restful Mind Support
- » Simply Adrenal
- » Simply Cardio
- » Simply Hypothalamus

- » Simply Liver
- » Simply Lung
- » Simply Mammary
- » Simply Orchic
- » Simply Ovary
- » Simply Pancreas
- » Simply Parotid
- » Simply Spleen
- » Simply Thymus
- » Simply Thyroid
- » Simply Uterus
- » Thymo Immune
- » Thymus EMG
- » Thyroid EMG

Glandulars, Enzomorphogens

- » Hypothalamus EMG
- » Pituitary EMG
- » Thymus EMG
- » Thyroid EMG

Glucoamylase

- » Biofilm Detox
- » Digesti-Pan

Glucosamine Sulfate (in Trachea)

- » Advanced Joint Complex
- » Complete Brain Health
- » Complete Eye Health

Glycyrrhiza

- » Vira-Chron

Goat's Rue

- » Gluco-Sugar Balance

Grape Seed/Skin Extract

- » Advanced Joint Complex
- » Complete Brain Health
- » Libida-Life

Grapefruit Seed Extract

- » Biofilm Detox
- » Para-Dysbio-Zyme

Grapes

- » Catalyst Complex
- » Vitamin & Mineral Shake

Guggul Gum

- » Cholester-Right

Gymnema Sylvestre

- » Gluco-Sugar-Balance

H

Hawthorn

- » Cardio-Power
- » Cholester-Right
- » CoQ10-Cardio

Heart, Bovine

- √ **Simply Cardio**
- √ **Cardio-Power**
- » Intracellular Cough
- » Ligament Complex

Hemicellulase

- » Biofilm Detox

Hemp

- » Vitamin & Mineral Shake

Herring

- » Omega 3/EPA/DHA

Honey

- » Dento-Gums

Horsetail Herb

- » Advanced Joint Complex
- » Cal-Mag Complex

Hydrochloric Acid

- » Calcium Lactate +
- » Digesti-Pan
- » Nerve Chex B

Hypothalamus, Bovine

- √ **Simply Hypothalamus**
- √ **Hypothalamus EMG**
- » Anxie-Tone
- » High Stress Adrenal
- » Intracellular Cough
- » Nerve Chex B
- » Restful Mind Support

I

Icelandic Moss

- » Arginase Bladder
- » Complete Ear Health
- » Intracellular Cough
- » Ligament Complex
- » Probio-Zyme-YST
- » Vegetarian Thyro

Indole-3-Carbinol (in Broccoli)

- » Complete Eye Health
- » Metabolic Thyro

Inositol, Food

- √ **Inositol Complex**
- » Anxie-Tone
- » B Stress Complex
- » Complete Brain Health
- » High Stress Adrenal
- » Ligament Complex
- » Vitamin-Mineral

Intestinal Tissue

- » Intestinal Support

Invertase

- » Digesti-Pan
- » Green Vegetable Alkalizer
- » Pro-Enzymes

Iodine, Food

- » Anxie-Tone
- » Beet-Food Plus
- » Cholester-Right
- » High Stress Adrenal

» Land and Sea Minerals
» Metabolic Thyro
» Mineral Transport
» Nerve Chex B
» Vegetarian Adrenal
» Vegetarian Thyro
» Vitamin-Mineral
» Vitamin & Mineral Shake

Iron, Food

√ **Hematic Formula**
» Vitamin-Mineral

Isoflavones *(in Red Clover)*

» Feminine Advantage

J

Jerusalem Artichoke

» Probio-Zyme-YST

Juniper Berries

» Intracellular Cough

K

Kelp, Atlantic

» Anxie-Tone
» Cholester-Right

Kelp, Thallus/ Sea Vegetables

» High Stress Adrenal
» Land and Sea Minerals
» Metabolic Thyro
» Mineral Transport
» Nerve Chex B
» Vegetarian Adrenal
» Vegetarian Thyro

Kidney, Bovine

√ **Kidney Support**
» A-C-P Complex
» Arginase Bladder
» Beet-Food Plus
» Catalyst Complex
» Ligament Complex

L

L-Arginine

» Libida-Life

L-Carnosine

» Complete Brain Health

L- Cysteine

▪ *Cysteine is naturally in all products that contain glandulars, as well as those with Saccharomyces cerevisiae.*

L-Glutamine

▪ *Glutamine is found in all glandular products.*

L-Methionine

» Complete Brain Health
» Detox-N-Cleanse *(in Sesame Seeds)*
▪ *L-Methionine is also found in all glandular products.*

L-Ornithine

» Libida-Life

L-Phenylalanine

» Vegetarian Tyrosine *and all glandular containing products.*

L-Serine

» Vegetarian Adrenal

L-Tryptophan

» Restful Mind Support
» Vegetarian Tryptophan

L-Tyrosine

» Anxie-Tone
» Complete Brain Health
» High Stress Adrenal
» Metabolic Thyro

» Vegetarian Adrenal
» Vegetarian Thyro
» Vegetarian Tyrosine

Lactase

» Digesti-Pan
» Green Vegetable Alkalizer
» Pro-Enzymes
» Vitamin & Mineral Shake

Lactobacillus acidophilus

» Pro-Enzymes
» Probio-Zyme-YST

Lactobacillus Bulgaricus *(Biogurt)*

» Catalyst Complex
» Magnesium Complex
» Mineral Transport
» Parathyroid Plus

Lactose

» Probio-Zyme-YST

Lecithin, Sunflower

» A-C-P Complex
» Beet-Food Plus
» Catalyst Complex
» Complete Brain Health
» Intracellular Cough
» Ligament Complex

Lemon Balm

» Restful Mind Support

Licorice Root

» Dento-Gums

Lion's Mane

» Lith-Mag-Forte
» Organic Mushrooms

Linseed

▪ *See Flaxseed*

Lipase

» Digesti-Pan
» Green Vegetable Alkalizer
» Para-Dysbio-Zyme
» Pro-Enzymes
» Simply Pancreas
» Vitamin & Mineral Shake

Lipoic Acid

» Complete Brain Health

Lithium

» Lith-Mag-Forte

Liver, Bovine

√ Simply Liver
√ Liva-DeTox & Support
» Arginase Bladder
» Beet-Food Plus
» Cardio-Power
» Catalyst Complex
» Complete Smell & Taste
» Conga-Immune
» GB Support
» Intestinal Support
» Intracellular Cough
» Kidney Support
» Ligament Complex
» Metabolic Thyro
» Migratrol
» Nerve Chex B
» Thymo-Immune

Lonicera

» Vira-Chron

Lung

» Simply Lung

Lutein

» Complete Eye Health

Lycopene

» Complete Eye Health
» Vegetarian Adrenal

Lymph, Bovine

» Conga-Immune
» Intestinal Support
» Intracellular Cough

Lysozyme

» Biofilm Detox

M

Maca

» Libida-Life
» Masculine Advantage

Magnesium, Food

√ Magnesium Complex
» Advanced Joint Complex
» Beet-Food Plus
» Cal-Mag Complex
» Calcium Lactate +
» Catalyst Complex
» Complete Smell & Taste
» Inflam-Enzymes
» Lith-Mag-Forte
» Migratrol
» Mineral Transport
» Nerve Chex B
» Parathyroid Plus

Magnolia

» Vira-Chron

Maitaki Mushroom

» A-C-P Complex
» Catalyst Complex

Maltase

» Green Vegetable Alkalizer
» Vitamin & Mineral Shake

Mammary, Bovine

» Simply Mammary

Manganese, Food

» Cal-Mag Complex

» Inflam-Enzymes
» Ligament Complex
» Nerve Chex B
» Pro-Enzymes
» Vitamin-Mineral
» Vitamin & Mineral Shake

Medulla, Bovine

» Complete Brain Health

Milk Thistle

» Beet-Food Plus
» Biofilm Detox
» Herbal Antioxidant
» Libida-Life
» Liva-DeTox & Support

Molybdenum, Food

» Vitamin-Mineral
» Vitamin & Mineral Shake

Monk Fruit

» Catalyst Complex

Monosaccharides, Essential All

» Metabolic Thyro

Moutan

» Vira-Chron

Mushroom Blend

» Catalyst Complex

Muira-Puama

» Masculine Advantage

N

N-Aceytl-L-Cysteine

» Complete Ear Health
» Gluco-Sugar-Balance

Nattokinase

» Nattokinase

Neem Oil

- » Dento-Gums

Nettle Leaf

- » Vira-Chron

Niacinamide, Food (Vitamin B-3)

- » Anxie-Tone
- » B Stress Complex
- » High Stress Adrenal
- » Migratrol
- » Nerve Chex B
- » Vitamin-Mineral
- » Vitamin & Mineral Shake

O

Okra (fruit)

- » Digesti-Pan
- » Inositol Complex

Olive Leaf Extract

- » Probio-Zyme-YST
- » Vira-Bac-YST
- » Vira-Chron

Omega 3

- √ Omega 3/EPA/DHA
- » Complete Brain Health
- » Complete Eye Health
- » Feminine Advantage

Orange, Fruit

- » Aller-Lung Support
- » C Complex
- » Cal-Mag Complex
- » Herbal Antioxidant
- » Hematic Formula
- » High Stress Adrenal
- » Vitamin-Mineral

Orchic, Bovine

- √ Simply Orchic
- √ Masculine Advantage
- » Beet-Food Plus
- » Nerve Chex B

Oregano Leaf

- » Biofilm Detox
- » Probio-Zyme-YST
- » Vira-Bac-YST
- » Vira-Chron

Ovary, Bovine

- √ Simply Ovary
- » Feminine Advantage
- » Restful Mind Support

Ox Bile, Bovine

- » GB Support
- » Intestinal Support

P

Pancreas, Bovine

- √ Simply Pancreas
- √ Digesti-Pan
- » Complete Brain Health
- » Intestinal Support
- » Kidney Support

Pantothenate, Food (Vitamin B-5)

- » Anxie-Tone
- » B Stress Complex
- » High Stress Adrenal
- » Vegetarian Adrenal
- » Vitamin-Mineral
- » Vitamin & Mineral Shake

Papain

- » Inflam-Enzymes

Para-Amino Benzoic Acid (PABA)

- » Ligament Complex
- » Nerve Chex B

Parathyroid, Bovine

- » Intracellular Cough
- » Parathyroid Plus

Parotid, Bovine

- √ Simply Parotid
- » Anxie-Tone
- » Complete Smell & Taste
- » Restful Mind Support
- » Thymo-Immune

Parsley Leaf

- » Arginase Bladder
- » Catalyst Complex
- » Green Vegetable Alkalizer
- » Mineral Transport
- » Vitamin & Mineral Shake

Passion Flower

- » Anxie-Tone
- » Intracellular Cough

Pectinase

- » Biofilm Detox

Peppermint/ Peppermint Leaf

- » Calcium Lactate +
- » Vitamin & Mineral Shake

Pepsin

- » Digesti-Pan

Peptidase

- » Biofilm Detox

Phellodendron

- » Vira-Chron

Phosphorus, Food

- All FOOD products contain phosphorus.

Pineal, Ovine or Bovine

- » Intracellular Cough
- » Restful Mind Support

Pituitary, Bovine

- √ Pituitary EMG

- » Complete Brain Health
- » Intracellular Cough
- » Metabolic Thyro
- » Migratrol
- » Restful Mind Support

Policosanol

- » Cholester-Right

Polysaccharides, Plant

- » Metabolic Thyro

Pomegranate

- » Cholester-Right

Potassium, Food

- • *All Food products contain potassium, but highest percentage is probably in:*
- » Green Vegetable Alkalizer

Psyllum

- » Probio-Zyme-YST

Proanthocyanidins

- » Advanced Joint Complex
- » Complete Brain Health

Probiotics

- » Pro-Enzymes
- » Probio-Zyme-YST
- » Vitamin & Mineral Shake

Prostate, Bovine

- √ **Masculine Advantage**
- » Beet-Food Plus

Proteolytic Enzymes/ Protease

- » Biofilm Detox
- » Digesti-Pan
- » Green Vegetable Alkalizer
- » Pro-Enzymes
- » Vitamin & Mineral Shake

Pumpkin Seeds

- » Arginase Bladder
- » Pro-Enzymes
- » Vegetarian Tyrosine
- » Zinc Complex

Q

Quercitin

- » Aller-Lung Support

R

Red Clover Blossom

- » Feminine Advantage
- » Kidney Support

Red Peony Root

- » Vira-Chron

Reishi Mushroom

- » Organic Mushrooms

Resveratrol

- » Libida-Life

Riboflavin, Food (*Vitamin B-2*)

- » Anxie-Tone
- » B Stress Complex
- » Catalyst Complex
- » High Stress Adrenal
- » Migratrol
- » Nerve Chex B
- » Vitamin-Mineral
- » Vitamin & Mineral Shake

Ribonucleic Acid (*RNA*)

- » Complete Brain Health
- » Ligament Complex

Rhizopus Oryzae

- » Arginase Bladder

Rosemary *(Flower & Leaf)*

- » Complete Eye Health
- » Herbal Antioxidant

Rutin *(in Buckwheat)*

- » A-C-P Complex
- » Arginase Bladder
- » Conga-Immune
- » Kidney Support
- » Vira-Bac-YST

S

Saccharomyces Cerevisiae

- » A-C-P Complex
- » Advanced Joint Complex
- » Anxie-Tone
- » B Stress Complex
- » Beet-Food Plus
- » Cal-Mag Complex
- » Calcium Complex
- » Cardio-Power
- » Catalyst Complex
- » Choline Complex
- » Complete Ear Health
- » Complete Eye Health
- » Complete Smell & Taste
- » Conga-Immune
- » D Complex
- » Gluco-Sugar-Balance
- » Hematic Formula
- » Herbal Antioxidant
- » High Stress Adrenal
- » Inflam-Enzymes
- » Inositol Complex
- » Land and Sea Minerals
- » Ligament Complex
- » Masculine Advantage
- » Metabolic Thyro
- » Migratrol
- » Parathyroid Plus
- » Probio-Zyme-YST
- » Selenium E
- » Complete Brain Health
- » Vegetarian Adrenal
- » Vegetarian Thyro
- » Vitamin-Mineral
- » Vitamin & Mineral Shake

» Vitamin B-6, B-12 & Folate
» Zinc Complex

Saw Palmetto Berry

» Masculine Advantage

Schisandra Fruit

» Herbal Antioxidant

Scullcap

» Metabolic Thyro

Selenium, Food

√ **Selenium E**
» Cardio-Power
» Complete Brain Health
» Complete Eye Health
» Herbal Antioxidant
» Libida-Life
» Masculine Advantage
» Vitamin-Mineral
» Vitamin & Mineral Shake

Serrapeptase

» Inflam-Enzymes
» Biofilm Detox

Sesame Seeds

» Detox-N-Cleanse

Shiitake Mushroom

» Biofilm Detox
» Catalyst Complex
» Choline Complex
» Conga-Immune
» D Complex
» Ligament Complex
» Organic Mushrooms

Silicon, Food

» Advanced Joint Complex
» Cal-Mag Complex
» Vitamin-Mineral
» Vitamin & Mineral Shake

Silymarin *(in Milk Thistle)*

• *See Milk Thistle*

Slippery Elm

» Detox-N-Cleanse

Sodium, Food *(in Kelp)*

» Anxie-Tone
» Cholester-Right
» High Stress Adrenal
» Land and Sea Minerals
» Metabolic Thyro
» Mineral Transport
» Nerve Chex B
» Vegetarian Adrenal
» Vegetarian Thyro
» Vitamin & Mineral Shake

Spinach

» Cal-Mag Complex
» Calcium Complex
» Green Vegetable Alkalizer
» Magnesium Complex
» Vitamin & Mineral Shake

Spirulina

» Green Vegetable Alkalizer
» Vitamin & Mineral Shake

Spleen, Bovine

√ **Simply Spleen**
» Calcium Lactate +
» Catalyst Complex
» Conga-Immune
» Dento-Gums
» Digesti-Pan
» Intracellular Cough
» Ligament Complex
» Liva-DeTox & Support
» Nerve Chex B
» Thymo-Immune

Stevia

» Vitamin & Mineral Shake

Stinging Nettles

» Aller-Lung Support
» Masculine Advantage
» Vira-Chron

Strawberry

» Catalyst Complex
» Dento-Gums

Suma

» Masculine Advantage

Sunflower Lecithin

• *See Lecithin, Sunflower*

Superoxide Dismutase *(SOD)*

» A-C-P Complex
» Advanced Joint Complex
» Anxie-Tone
» B Stress Complex
» Beet-Food Plus
» Cal-Mag Complex
» Calcium Complex
» Cardio-Power
» Catalyst Complex
» Choline Complex
» Complete Brain Health
» Complete Ear Health
» Complete Eye Health
» Complete Smell & Taste
» Conga-Immune
» D Complex
» Gluco-Sugar-Balance
» Hematic Formula
» Herbal Antioxidant
» High Stress Adrenal
» Inflam-Enzymes
» Inositol Complex
» Magnesium Complex
» Masculine Advantage
» Metabolic Thyro
» Migratrol
» Parathyroid Plus
» Probio-Zyme-YST
» Selenium E
» Vegetarian Adrenal
» Vegetarian Thyro
» Vitamin-Mineral
» Vitamin & Mineral Shake
» Vitamin B-6, B-12 & Folate
» Zinc Complex

Sweet Violet

» Probio-Zyme-YST

Sweet Wormwood

» Para-Dysbio-Zyme

T

Thiamin, Food
(*Vitamin B-1*)

» Anxie-Tone
» B Stress Complex
» Catalyst Complex
» High Stress Adrenal
» Nerve Chex B
» Vitamin-Mineral
» Vitamin & Mineral Shake

Thyme

» Aller-Lung Support

Thymus, Bovine

√ **Simply Thymus**
√ **Thymo-Immune**
√ **Thymus EMG**
» Anxie-Tone
» Complete Ear Health
» Conga-Immune
» Intracellular Cough

Thyroid, Bovine

√ **Simply Thyroid**
√ **Thyroid EMG**
» Intracellular Cough
» Metabolic Thyro
» Migratrol

Tomatoes

» Complete Eye Health
» Vegetarian Adrenal

Tongue, Goat/Ovine

» Complete Smell & Taste

Trachea, Bovine

» Advanced Joint Complex
» Complete Brain Health

» Complete Eye Health
» Intracellular Cough

Trypsin, Bovine

» Hypothalamus EMG
» Pituitary EMG
» Simply Pancreas
» Thymus EMG
» Thyroid EMG

Turkey Tail

» Organic Mushrooms

Turmeric Rhizome/Root

√ **Turmeric-Boswellia C**
» Cholester-Right
» Herbal Antioxidant
» Masculine Advantage

U

Ubiquinone

» CoQ10-Cardio
» Vitamin-Mineral

Uña De Gato

▪ *See Cat's Claw*

Uterus, Bovine

√ **Simply Uterus**
» Feminine Advantage

Uva Ursi

» Intracellular Cough

V

Vanadium, Food

» Gluco-Sugar-Balance
» Vitamin-Mineral

Vanilla

» Vitamin & Mineral Shake

Vitamin A (*Alpha/ Betacarotene*)

√ **Complete Eye Health**
» A-C-P Complex
» Beet-Food Plus
» Catalyst Complex
» Herbal Antioxidant
» Ligament Complex
» Vitamin-Mineral
» Vitamin & Mineral Shake

Vitamin B Complex

√ **B Stress Complex**
√ **Vitamin B-6, B-12 & Folate**
» Anxie-Tone
» High Stress Adrenal
» Nerve Chex B
» Vitamin-Mineral
» Vitamin & Mineral Shake

Vitamin B-1, Food
(*Thiamin*)

√ **B Stress Complex**
» Anxie-Tone
» Catalyst Complex
» High Stress Adrenal
» Nerve Chex B
» Vitamin-Mineral
» Vitamin-Mineral B

Vitamin B-2, Food
(*Riboflavin*)

√ **B Stress Complex**
» Anxie-Tone
» Catalyst Complex
» High Stress Adrenal
» Migratrol
» Nerve Chex B
» Vitamin-Mineral
» Vitamin & Mineral Shake

Vitamin B-3, Food
(*Niacinamide*)

√ **B Stress Complex**
» Anxie-Tone
» High Stress Adrenal
» Migratrol
» Nerve Chex B

» Vitamin-Mineral
» Vitamin & Mineral Shake

Vitamin B-5, Food (Pantothenate)

√ **B Stress Complex**
» Anxie-Tone
» High Stress Adrenal
» Vegetarian Adrenal
» Vitamin-Mineral
» Vitamin & Mineral Shake

Vitamin B-6, Food

√ **Vitamin B-6, B-12 & Folate**
√ **B Stress Complex**
» Anxie-Tone
» Beet-Food Plus
» Cardio-Power
» Catalyst Complex
» Complete Brain Health
» Hematic Formula
» High Stress Adrenal
» Nerve Chex B
» Vegetarian Adrenal
» Vegetarian Thyro
» Vitamin-Mineral
» Vitamin & Mineral Shake

Vitamin B-7, Food (Biotin)

√ **B Stress Complex**
» Anxie-Tone
» Vitamin-Mineral
» Vitamin & Mineral Shake

Vitamin B-9, Food (Folate)

√ **Vitamin B-6, B-12 & Folate**
√ **B Stress Complex**
» Anxie-Tone
» Cardio-Power
» Complete Brain Health
» Hematic Formula
» High Stress Adrenal
» Vegetarian Adrenal
» Vegetarian Thyro
» Vitamin-Mineral
» Vitamin & Mineral Shake

Vitamin B-12, Food

√ **Vitamin B-6, B-12 & Folate**

√ **B Stress Complex**
» Anxie-Tone
» Cardio-Power
» Complete Brain Health
» Hematic Formula
» High Stress Adrenal
» Ligament Complex
» Nerve Chex B
» Vegetarian Adrenal
» Vegetarian Thyro
» Vitamin-Mineral
» Vitamin & Mineral Shake

Vitamin "B-17"

» Complete Brain Health
» Para-Dysbio-Zyme
» Vira-Bac-YST

Vitamin C, Food

√ **C Complex**
√ **Turmeric-Boswellia C**
» A-C-P Complex
» Advanced Joint Complex
» Aller-Lung Support
» Anxie-Tone
» Arginase Bladder
» Cal-Mag Complex
» Cardio-Power
» Catalyst Complex
» Cholester-Right
» Complete Brain Health
» Complete Ear Health
» Complete Eye Health
» Conga-Immune
» CoQ10-Cardio
» Dento-Gums
» Detox-N-Cleanse
» Hematic Formula
» Herbal Antioxidant
» High Stress Adrenal
» Inflam-Enzymes
» Intracellular Cough
» Kidney Support
» Ligament Complex
» Nerve Chex B
» Thymo-Immune
» Vegetarian Adrenal
» Vitamin-Mineral
» Vitamin & Mineral Shake

Vitamin D, Food

√ **D Complex**
» Advanced Joint Complex
» Cal-Mag Complex
» Catalyst Complex
» Ligament Complex
» Parathyroid Plus
» Vitamin-Mineral
» Vitamin & Mineral Shake

Vitamin E, Food

√ **Selenium E**
√ **Wheat Germ Oil E**
» A-C-P Complex
» Beet-Food Plus
» Cardio-Power
» Complete Brain Health

» Complete Eye Health
» Herbal Antioxidant
» Ligament Complex
» Masculine Advantage
» Omega 3/EPA/DHA
» Vitamin-Mineral
» Vitamin & Mineral Shake

Vitamin "F" (Essentially Fatty Acids)

» Beet-Food Plus
» Complete Brain Health
» Complete Eye Health
» Feminine Advantage
» Ligament Complex
» Masculine Advantage
» Migratrol
» Omega 3/EPA/DHA
» Wheat Germ Oil E

Vitamin "G" (Riboflavin)

√ **B Stress Complex**
» Anxie-Tone
» Catalyst Complex
» High Stress Adrenal
» Migratrol
» Nerve Chex B
» Vitamin-Mineral
» Vitamin & Mineral Shake

Vitamin "H" (Biotin)

√ **B Stress Complex**
- » Anxie-Tone
- » Vitamin-Mineral
- » Vitamin & Mineral Shake

Vitamin K, Food

- » Cal-Mag Complex
- » Green Vegetable Alkalizer
- » Vitamin-Mineral
- » Vitamin & Mineral Shake

Vitamin "P" (Bioflavonoids)

- » A-C-P Complex
- » Advanced Joint Complex
- » Aller-Lung Support
- » Anxie-Tone
- » Arginase Bladder
- » C Complex
- » Cal-Mag Complex
- » Cardio-Power
- » Catalyst Complex
- » Cholester-Right
- » Complete Brain Health
- » Complete Ear Health
- » Complete Eye Health
- » Conga-Immune
- » CoQ10-Cardio
- » Dento-Gums
- » Detox-N-Cleanse
- » Hematic Formula
- » Herbal Antioxidant
- » High Stress Adrenal
- » Inflam-Enzymes
- » Intracellular Cough
- » Kidney Support
- » Ligament Complex
- » Nerve Chex B
- » Thymo-Immune
- » Vegetarian Adrenal
- » Vitamin-Mineral
- » Vitamin & Mineral Shake

Vitex

- » Vira-Chron

W

Watercress

- » Green Vegetable Alkalizer
- » Vitamin & Mineral Shake

Wheat Germ (Defatted)

√ **Wheat Germ Oil E**
- » A-C-P Complex
- » Beet-Food Plus
- » Catalyst Complex
- » Dento-Gums
- » Ligament Complex
- » Nerve Chex B
- » Probio-Zyme-YST

Wheat Germ Oil

√ **Wheat Germ Oil E**

Wheatgrass

- » A-C-P Complex
- » Catalyst Complex
- » Detox-N-Cleanse
- » Green Vegetable Alkalizer
- » Ligament Complex
- » Vitamin & Mineral Shake

Wild Yam Root (Mexican)

- » Dento-Gums
- » Feminine Advantage

Wolfberries

- » Complete Eye Health

X

Xanthium

- » Vira-Chron

Y

Yucca

- » Advanced Joint Complex

Z

Zeaxanthin

- » Complete Eye Health

Zinc

√ **Zinc Complex**
- » Advanced Joint Complex
- » Complete Ear Health
- » Complete Eye Health
- » Complete Smell & Taste
- » Conga-Immune
- » Herbal Antioxidant
- » High Stress Adrenal
- » Libida-Life
- » Masculine Advantage
- » Probio-Zyme-YST
- » Vegetarian Thyro
- » Vitamin-Mineral
- » Vitamin & Mineral Shake

More Doctors' Research Support Literature and Educational Items

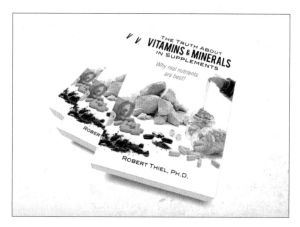

The TRUTH About VITAMINS & MINERALS in SUPPLEMENTS

Do you know what vitamins and minerals do for the human body? Are there some forms of vitamins and minerals better than others? Many people have wrongly assumed that vitamin and mineral formulas they buy are natural and are the same as vitamins and minerals as found in food. This highly referenced book explains the biological advantages of food vitamins and minerals as well as their superiority. It also explains what most "so-called natural" vitamins and minerals are actually made from. This is a must have book for people interested in health so they do not make the common mistakes 99% of people who take vitamin and mineral supplements do.

Brochures

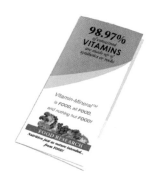

Vitamin-Mineral Brochure

98.97% of consumed Vitamins are made up of synthetics or rocks, Food Research Products are FOOD, all FOOD, and nothing but FOOD!

Unlike synthetic products, our supplements contain the enzymes and peptides found in living foods. The vitamins and minerals are cold-processed. Our vitamin and mineral products stay below 100°F, hence they are considered to be "raw."

This brochure will show you "How To Read Your Vitamin Labels."

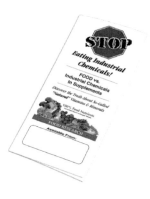

STOP Chemicals Brochure

Should Your Vitamin and Mineral Supplements Be Made from 100% FOOD or Industrial Chemicals?

Amazingly, 98.97% of people who take so-called 'natural' vitamin products are taking vitamins that are composed of petroleum-derivatives, oils, hydrogenated acetone-processed sugars, and/or irradiated animal fats. And nearly all of the people who take mineral products are taking minerals which are crushed rocks processed with industrial chemicals (like those shown in this brochure).

In this brochure, discover the Truth About So-Called "Natural" Vitamins & Minerals.

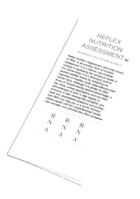

Reflex Nutrition Assessment (RNA) Brochure

Reflex Nutrition Assessment, otherwise known as RNA, is an ancillary form of nutrition assessment. It is a natural, non-invasive method of assessing the nutritional needs of the human body. It is a technique used to assess nutrition status by observing the response of muscles under externally-provided human force.

Although it is similar to other forms of muscle testing (deltoid kinesiology), it has many unique applications and has been demonstrated to have a high degree of accuracy. If after reading this pamphlet, you have any unanswered questions concerning how RNA can help you or a family member, please speak with the doctor/licensed health care provider who provided this RNA pamphlet.

The Truth About Vitamins in Nutritional Supplements

ABSTRACT: *Even though natural health professionals agree that humans should not try to consume petroleum derivatives or hydrogenated sugars, most seem to overlook this fact when vitamin supplementation is involved. This paper explains some of the biochemical reasons that food vitamins are superior for humans. It also explains what substances are commonly used to make vitamins in supplements. Furthermore, it explains some of the advantages of food vitamins over the non-food vitamins that are commonly available.*

For decades the 'natural' health industry has been touting thousands of vitamin supplements. The truth is that most vitamins in supplements are made of or processed with petroleum derivatives or hydrogenated sugars [1-5], hence they are synthetic. Even though they are often called natural, most non-food vitamins are isolated substances which are crystalline in structure [1]. Vitamins naturally in food are not crystalline and never isolated. Non-food vitamins are isolates, which means that they are individual chemicals lacking substances that real foods contain. Vitamins found in any real food are chemically and structurally different from those commonly found in 'natural vitamin' formulas. Food vitamins contain a matrix of substances which improve bioavailability and safety. Since they are different, naturally-oriented people should consider non-food vitamins as vitamin analogues (imitations) and not actually vitamins. Whether sold retail or wholesale, nearly all companies sell synthetic vitamins.

The standards of naturopathy agreed to in 1947 (at the Golden Jubilee Congress) included the statements, "Naturopathy does not make use of synthetic or inorganic vitamins...Naturopathy makes use of the healing properties of...natural foods, organic vitamins" [5]. Even back in the 1940's, professionals interested in natural health recognized the value of food, over non-food, vitamins. Also, it should be mentioned that naturopathic definition of organic back then was similar to the official US government definition today--why does this need to be stated? Because one pseudo-naturopath once told this researcher that a particular brand of synthetic vitamins contained "organic vitamins," because a sales representative had told him so. Sadly, that sales representative either intentionally gave out false information or gave out misleading information--misleading because by its 'scientific' definition, the term 'organic' can mean that it is a carbon containing substance. By that definition all petroleum derivatives (hydro-carbons) are organic. This is false, because those type of vitamins are not organic from the true naturopathic, or even the U.S. government's, perspective.

Officially, according to mainstream science, "Vitamins are organic substances that are essential in small amounts for the health, growth, reproduction, and maintenance of one or more animal species, which must be included in the diet since they cannot be synthesized at all or in sufficient quantity in the body. Each vitamin performs a specific function; hence one cannot replace another. Vitamins originate primarily in plant tissues" [6]. Isolated non-food 'vitamins' (often called 'natural' or USP or pharmaceutical grade) are not naturally "included in the diet", do not necessarily "originate primarily in plant tissues", and cannot fully replace all natural vitamin activities. As a natural health professional, you should be able to read and interpret, even misleading supplement labels. For those who are unsure, hopefully this article will provide sufficient information to determine if vitamin tablets are food or imitations.

What is Your Vitamin Really?

Most vitamins in supplements are petroleum extracts, coal tar derivatives, and chemically processed sugar (plus sometimes industrially processed fish oils), with other acids and industrial chemicals (such as formaldehyde) used to process them [1-5].

Synthetic vitamins were originally developed because they cost less [7]. Assuming the non-food product does not contain fish oils, most synthetic, petroleum-derived, supplements will call their products 'vegetarian', not because they are from plants, but because they are not from animals.

Most USP 'vitamins' are chemical analogues of vitamins, meaning that they are in a chemical form that some scientists say is similar to the forms found in nature. Analogues are NOT the real thing.

Table 1. Composition of Food and Non-Food Vitamins [1-10]

Vitamin	Food Nutrient*	Natural' Vitamin Analogue & Some Process Chemicals
Vitamin A/Betacarotene	Carrots	Methanol, benzene, petroleum esters; acetylene; refined oils
Vitamin B-1	Nutritional yeast, rice bran	Coal tar derivatives, hydrochloric acid; acetonitrole with ammonia
Vitamin B-2	Nutritional yeast, rice bran	Synthetically produced with 2N acetic acid
Vitamin B-3	Nutritional yeast, rice bran	Coal tar derivatives, 3-cyanopyridine; ammonia and acid
Vitamin B-5	Nutritional yeast, rice bran	Condensing isobutyraldehyde with formaldehyde
Vitamin B-6	Nutritional yeast, rice bran	Petroleum ester & hydrochloric acid with formaldehyde
Vitamin B-8	Nutritional yeast, rice bran	Phytin hydrolyzed with calcium hydroxide and sulfuric acid
Vitamin B-9	Nutritional yeast, rice bran	Processed with petroleum derivatives and acids; acetylene
Vitamin B-12	Nutritional yeast	Cobalamins reacted with cyanide
Vitamin 'B-x' PABA	Nutritional yeast	Coal tar oxidized with nitric acid (from ammonia)
Choline	Nutritional yeast, rice bran	Ethylene and ammonia with HCL or tartaric acid
Vitamin C	Acerola cherries, citrus fruits	Hydrogenated sugar processed with acetone
Vitamin D	Nutritional yeast, mushrooms	Irradiated animal fat/cattle brains or solvently extracted
Vitamin E	Nutritional yeast, vegetable oils	Trimethylhydroquinone with isophytol; refined oils
Vitamin H	Nutritional yeast, rice bran	Biosynthetically produced
Vitamin K	Alfalfa	Coal tar derivative; produced with p-allelic-nickel

* Note: Some companies use liver extracts as a source for vitamins A and/or D, and at least one company has a herring oil product supplying some vitamin E. No company this researcher is aware of whose products are made out of 100% food use animal products in any of their multiple vitamins. Some companies also use brewer's yeast which is inferior to nutritional yeast in many ways (including the fact that it has not had the cell wall enzymatically processed to reduce possible sensitivities).

Read The Label to See the Chemical Differences!

Although many doctors have been taught that food and non-food vitamins have the same chemical composition, this is simply untrue for most vitamins. As shown in **table 2**, the chemical forms of food and synthetic nutrients are normally different.

Health professionals need to understand that there is no mandated definition of the term 'natural' when it comes to vitamins; just seeing that term on a label does not mean that the supplement contains only natural food substances. One of the best ways to tell whether or not a vitamin supplement contains natural vitamins as found in food is to know the chemical differences between food and non-food vitamins (sometimes called USP vitamins). Because they are not normally in the same chemical form as vitamins found in foods, non-food vitamins should be considered by natural health professionals as vitamin analogues (artificial imitations), and not actually as true vitamins for humans.

Table 2. Chemical Form of Food and Non-Food Vitamins [1-10]

Primary Chemical Vitamin Form in Food	Vitamin Analogue Chemical Form (Often Called Natural*)
Vitamin A/Betacarotene; retinyl esters; mixed carotenoids	Vitamin A acetate; vitamin A palmitate; betacarotene (isolated)
Vitamin B-1; thiamin pyrophosphate (food)	Thiamin mononitrate; thiamin hydrochloride; thiamin HCL
Vitamin B-2; riboflavin, multiple forms (food)	Riboflavin (isolated); USP vitamin B2
Vitamin B-3; niacinamide (food)	Niacin (isolated); niacinamide (isolated)
Vitamin B-5; pantothenate (food)	Pantothenic acid; calcium pantothenate; panthenol
Vitamin B-6; 5'0 (beta-D) pyridoxine	Pyridoxine hydrochloride; pyridoxine HCL
Vitamin B-9; folate	Folic acid
Vitamin B-12; methylcobalamin; deoxyadenosylcobalamin	Cyanocobalamin; hydroxycobalamin
Choline (food); phosphatidyl choline (food)	Choline chloride; choline bitartrate
Vitamin C; ascorbate (food); dehydroascorbate	Ascorbic acid; most mineral ascorbates(i.e. sodium ascorbate)
Vitamin D; mixed forms, primarily D3 (food)	Vitamin D1 (isolated); Vitamin D2 (isolated); Vitamin D3 (isolated)
Vitamin D; mixed forms, primarily D3 (food)	Vitamin D1 (isolated); Vitamin D2 (isolated); Vitamin D3 (isolated)
	Vitamin D4; ergosterol (isolated); cholecalciferol (isolated); lumisterol
Vitamin E; RRR-alpha-tocopherol (food)	Vitamin E acetate; Mixed tocopherols; all-rac-alpha-tocopherol; d-l--alpha-tocopherol; d-alpha-tocopherol (isolated); dl-alpha-tocopheryl acetate; all acetate forms
Vitamin H; biotin	All non-yeast or non-rice vegetarian biotin forms
Vitamin K; phylloquinone (food)	Vitamin K3; menadione; phytonadione; naphthoquinone; dihydro-vitamin K1

* Note: This list is not complete and new analogues are being developed all the time. Also the term "(isolated)" means that if the word "food" is not near the name of the substance, it is probably an isolate (normally crystalline in structure) and is not the same as the true vitamin found in food.

Read the label of any supplement to see if the product is truly 100% food. If even one USP vitamin analogue is listed, then the entire product is probably not food (normally it will be less than 5% food). Vitamin analogues are cheap (or not so cheap) imitations of vitamins found in foods.

Beware of any supplement label that says that its vitamins are vegetarian and contain no yeast. This researcher is unaware of any frequently used vegetarian non-yeast way to produce vitamin D or many of the B vitamins, therefore, if a label states that the product "contains no yeast" then in pretty much all cases, this demonstrates that the product is synthetic or contains items so isolated that they should not be considered to be food.

Saccharomyces cerevisiae (the primary yeast used in baking and brewing) is beneficial to humans and can help combat various infections [11], including, according to the German E monograph, *Candida albicans*. In the text, Medical Mycology John Rippon (Ph.D., Mycology, University of Chicago) wrote, "There are over 500 known species of yeast, all distinctly different. And although the so-called bad yeasts do exist, the controversy in the natural foods industry regarding yeast related to health problems which is causing many health-conscious people to eliminate all yeast products from their

diet is ridiculous. It should also be noted, that W. Crook, M.D., perhaps the nation's best known expert on Candida albicans, wrote, "yeasty foods don't encourage candida growth...Eating a yeast-containing food does not make candida organisms multiply" [12]. Some people, however, are allergic to the cell-wall of yeast [12] and concerned supplement companies which have nutrient-containing yeast normally have had the cell-wall enzymatically processed to reduce even this unlikely occurrence.

Food Vitamins are Superior to Non-Food Vitamins

Although many mainstream health professionals believe, "The body cannot tell whether a vitamin in the bloodstream came from an organically grown cantaloupe or from a chemist's laboratory" [13], this belief is quite misleading for several reasons.

• First, it seems to assume that the process of getting the amount of the vitamin into the bloodstream is the same (which is frequently not the case [3-10]).

• Secondly, scientists understand that particle size is an important factor in nutrient absorption even though particle size is not detected by chemical assessment.

• Thirdly, scientists also understand that, "The food factors that influence the absorption of nutrients relate not only to the nature of the nutrients themselves, but also their interaction with each other and with the nonabsorbable components of food" [14].

• Fourthly, "the physiochemical form of a nutrient is a major factor in bioavailability" (and food and non-food vitamins are not normally in the same form) [15].

• Fifthly, most non-food vitamins are crystalline in structure [1].

Published scientific research has concluded, "natural vitamins are nutritionally superior to synthetic ones" [8].

Food vitamins are in the physiochemical forms which the body recognizes, generally are not crystalline in structure, contain food factors that affect bioavailability, and appear to have smaller particle sizes *(see illustrations in table 3)*. This does not mean that non-food vitamins do not have any value (they clearly do), but it is important to understand that natural food complex vitamins have actually been shown to be better than isolated, non-food, vitamins (see table 4).

Electronic photos demonstrate that isolated USP vitamins have a crystalline appearance compared to vitamins in foods which have more of a rounded appearance (see table 3).

Natural Foods are produced as a result of living biological processes and nutrients in them appear to be contained in rounded food components. USP vitamins are the result of chemical processes which make them be, as well as appear, crystalline in form. The form that isolated crystallized chemical USP vitamins have, never happens in nature.

Table 3. Physical and Structural Differences

Electronic Photographs

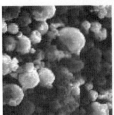 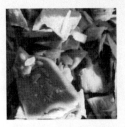 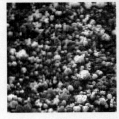 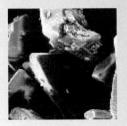

| Food Vitamin B-1 | USP Vitamin B-1 | Food Vitamin C | USP Vitamin C |

Even before these types of pictures were available, the late Dr. Royal Lee knew that food vitamin C was superior to ascorbic acid. "Dr. Lee felt it was not honest to use the name 'vitamin C' for ascorbic acid. That term 'should be reserved for the vitamin C COMPLEX'" [16]. Why then, according to the ingredients listed in a recent catalog, would a supplement company that Dr. Lee originally founded currently include ascorbic acid, inorganic mineral salts, and/or other isolated nutrients in the majority of its products? Dr. Lee, like the late Dr. Bernard Jensen [17], was also opposed to the use of other isolated, synthetic nutrients [16].

Dr Lee specifically wrote, "In fact, the Food & Drug laws seem to be suspended where synthetic imitations of good foods are concerned, and actually perverted to prosecute makers and sellers of real products...The synthetic product is always a simple chemical substance, while the natural is a complex mixture of related and similar materials...Pure natural Vitamin E was found three times as potent as pure synthetic Vitamin E. Of course the poisonous nature of the synthetic Vitamin D...is well established. WHY DO NOT THE PEOPLE AND MEDICAL MEN KNOW THESE FACTS? Is it because the commercial promoters of cheap imitation food and drug products spend enough money to stop the leaking out of information?" [18].

Food vitamins are superior. The human body is not intended to ultiize unnatural, synthethic, crystalline 'vitamins.'

Table 4. Comparison of Certain Biological Effects of Food and Non-Food Vitamins

Food Vitamin	Compared to USP/'Natural'/Non-Food Vitamins
Vitamin A	54% more absorbed into the blood [19]; also more complete, as scientists teach that vitamin A is not an isolate [20]
Vitamin B Complex	More effective in maintaining good health and liver function [21,22]
Vitamin B-1, Thiamin	38% more absorbed into the blood [19]
Vitamin B-2, Riboflavin	92% more retained in the liver [19]
Vitamin B-3, Niacinamide	3.94 times more absorbed into the blood [19]
Vitamin B-5, Pantothenate	57% more absorbed into the blood [19].
Vitamin B-6	2.54 times more absorbed into the blood [19].
Vitamin B-9, Folate	2.13 times more retained in the liver; more utilizable above 266mcg (Recommended Daily Intake is 400mcg) [23] and safer [24].
Vitamin B-12	2.56 times more absorbed into the blood [19]
Vitamin C	Over 15.6 times antioxidant effect [25]; 74% better absorbed into red blood cells [19]
Vitamin D	Over 10 times the antirachitic effect [26]
Vitamin E	Up to 4.0 times the free radical scavenging strength [27]
Vitamin H	Up to 100 times more biotin effect [1]
Vitamin K	Safer for children [28]

The difference is more than quantitative.

Let's take vitamin C for an example. Even if one were to take 3.2 times as much of the so-called natural, non-food, ascorbic acid as food vitamin C, although the antioxidant effects might be similar *in vitro*, the ascorbic acid still will not contain DHAA [1], nor will it ever have negative oxidative reductive potential (ORP). An *in vitro* study performed at this researcher's lab with a digital ORP meter demonstrated that a citrus food vitamin C has negative ORP, but that ascorbic acid had positive ORP [29].

It takes negative ORP to clean up oxidative damage [30], and since ascorbic acid has positive ORP (as well as positive redox potential [1]), it can never replace food vitamin C no matter what the quantity! Furthermore, foods which are high in vitamin C tend to have high Oxygen Radical Absorbance Capacity (ORAC, another test which measures the ability of foods and other compounds to subdue oxygen free radicals [25]). A US government study which compared the *in vivo* effects of a high vitamin C food (containing 80 mg of vitamin C) compared to about 15.6 times as much isolated ascorbic acid (1250 mg) found that the vitamin C-containing food produced the greatest increase in blood antioxidant levels (it is believed that bioflavonoids and other food factors are responsible) [25].

Furthermore, it is even possible isolated ascorbic acid only has *in vitro* and no *in vivo* antioxidant effects: "it has not been possible to show conclusively that higher than anti-scorbic intake of {SYNTHETIC} vitamin C has antioxidant clinical benefit" [31]. Why should people take supplemental synthetic ascorbic acid when it has NOT been proven to have significant antioxidant effects in humans?

"Cross sectional and longitudinal studies show that the occurrence of cardiovascular disease and cancer is inversely related to vitamin C intake… the protective effects seen in these studies are attributable to fruit and vegetable {FOOD} intake… In general, beneficial effects of supplemental {SYNTHETIC} vitamin C have been noted in small studies, while large well controlled studies have failed to show benefit" [31]. The other quantitative is that in humans, "Plasma is completely saturated in doses of 400 mg and higher daily producing a steady-state plasma concentration of 80 mm…

Tissues, however, saturate before plasma" [31]. De-emphasizing vitamin C containing foods by attempting to consume higher quantities of isolated ascorbic acid simply will not have the effects on plasma vitamin C levels, ORP, ORAC, or other health aspects that many consumers of isolated ascorbic acid hope it will [3,29,31].

No matter how much isolated ascorbic acid one takes orally:

1) *It will never saturate plasma and/or tissue vitamin C levels significantly more than can be obtained by consuming sufficient vitamin C containing foods.*

2) *It will never have negative ORP, thus can never 'clean-up' oxidative damage like food vitamin C can.*

3) *It will never have the free radical fighting capacity of food vitamin C.*

4) *It will never contain DHAA (the other 'half' of vitamin C) or the promoting food factors.*

5) *It will never have the same effect on health issues, such as aging and cardiovascular disease as high vitamin C foods can.*

6) *It will not ever be utilized the way food vitamin C is.*

7) *It will always be a synthetic.*

Let's take vitamin E as another example—the body has a specific liver transport for the type of vitamin E found in food [10]—it does not have this for the synthetic vitamin E forms (nor for the 'new' vitamin E analogues that are frequently marketed)—thus no amount of synthetic vitamin E can truly equal food vitamin E—the human body actually tries to rid itself of synthetic vitamin E as quickly as possible [32]. As another example, it should be understood that certain forms of vitamin analogues of B-6 [19], D [10], and biotin [1] have been shown to have almost no vitamin activity.

Fractionated, synthetic, vitamins do not replace all the natural function of food vitamins in the body. This is due to the fact that they are normally chemically and structurally different from vitamins found in foods (or vitamin supplements made up entirely of foods). They also do not have the naturally occurring food factors which are needed by the body.

Food Vitamins and Non-Food Vitamin Analogues

Vitamin A/Betacarotene

Vitamin A naturally exists in foods, but not as a single compound. Vitamin A primarily exists in the form of retinyl esters, and not retinol and betacarotene is always in the presence of mixed carotenoids with chlorophyll [10]. Vitamin A acetate is from methanol, it is a retinol which is crystalline in structure [1]. Vitamin A palmitate can be fish oil [1] or synthetically derived [2]; but once isolated it bears little resemblance to food and can be crystalline in structure [1,2]. Synthetic betacarotene is "prepared from condensing aldehyde (from acetone) with acetylene" [2]; "not much natural beta-carotene is available due to the high costs of production" [2].

"Beta-carotene has been found to have antioxidant effect *in vitro*...Whether {ISOLATED} beta-carotene has significant antioxidant effect *in vivo* is unclear" [33]. Carrots, a food high in betacarotene, do have high antioxidant ability [33,34]. Natural betacarotene, as found in foods, is composed of both all-trans and 9-cis isomers, while synthetic betacarotene is all-trans isomers [35]. Carrots, yellow and green leafy vegetables, and turmeric contain natural betacarotene along with multiple carotenoids. Natural betacarotene was found to significantly decrease serum conjugated diene levels for children exposed to high levels of irradiation, though it is not

known if synthetic betacarotene would provide similar benefits [35].

Regarding isolated betacarotene, "The data presented provide convincing evidence of the harmful properties of this compound if given alone to smokers, or to individuals exposed to environmental carcinogens, as a micronutrient supplement" [36]. "The three beta-carotene intervention trials: the Betacarotene and Retinol Efficacy Trial (CARET), Alpha-Tocopherol, Beta-Carotene Cancer Prevention Study (ATBC), and Physician's Health Study (PHS) have all pointed to a lack of effect of synthetic beta-carotene in decreasing cardiovascular disease or cancer risk in well-nourished populations. The potential contribution of beta-carotene supplementation to increased risk of lung cancer in smokers has been raised as a significant concern. The safety of synthetic beta-carotene supplements and the role of isomeric forms of beta-carotene (synthetic all-trans versus "natural" cis-trans isomeric mixtures)... have become topics of debate in the scientific and medical communities" [37]. Now, although the consumption of both synthetic betacarotene and food betacarotene raise serum vitamin A levels about the same, this obscures the fact that synthetic betacarotene tends to mainly increase serums all-trans betacarotene, while food betacarotene increases other forms as well [38].

It is possible that synthetic betacarotene can negatively affect vitamin E's antioxidant ability as a clinical study found, "These results support earlier findings for the protective effect of a-tocopherol against LDL oxidation, and suggest that beta-carotene participates as a prooxidant in the oxidative degradation of LDL under these conditions. Since high levels of alpha-tocopherol did not mitigate the prooxidative effect of beta-carotene, these results indicate that increased LDL beta-carotene may cancel the protective qualities of alpha-tocopherol" [39]. In a consumer-directed publication, Stephen Sinatra (M.D.) observes, "Research has shown that high doses of synthetic beta-carotene—the kind found in many popular brands—may actually increase your risk for lung cancer. Because at high levels it can become prooxidative—exactly the opposite of what you want...I've seen harmful effects (such as serious vision loss) in people who have taken up to 80,000 IU of beta-carotene per day. The bottom line is: Less is more when it comes to beta-carotene. To be safe I recommend between 12,500 and 25,000 IU of beta-carotene per day from food sources such as carrots" [40].

In my opinion, betacarotene in carrots, however, is safer than even Dr. Sinatra suggests (there is about 12,000 i.u. of betacarotene in one raw carrot). The reason for this is because betacarotene in carrots is attached to lipoproteins which appear to aid in preventing toxicity. Isolated USP betacarotene, even if it allegedly comes from "natural" sources, simply

does not have the attached lipoproteins or other potentially protective substances as found in foods like carrots.

While isolated synthesized vitamin A and polar bear livers have posed toxicity issues, this is simply not considered to be the case of any other food that is supplying vitamin A/beta-carotene [41,42]. An animal study concluded that Food vitamin A is probably less toxic than USP isolated form and was 1.54 times more absorbed into the blood [19]. Foods containing vitamin A and/or betacarotene are superior [8].

Vitamin B-1, Thiamin

Vitamin B-1 exists in food in the forms of thiamin pyrophosphate, thiamin monophosphate, and thiamin [10]. The non-food thiamin mononitrate is a coal tar derivative [4], never naturally found in the body [10], and is a crystalline isolate [1] (the same is true for thiamin hydrochloride and other chloride forms). Synthetic forms are often used in "food fortification" (where processing removes the naturally occurring thiamin) as they are cheaper and, in that context more stable. However, they are inferior

to naturally occurring thiamin forms [8,42]. "The nutritive value of straight-run white flour...has been found to be inferior to that of wholemeal flour, even when the defects of the former in protein, minerals and {SYNTHETIC} vitamin B1 have been corrected" [43]. An animal study found that Food vitamin B-1 was absorbed 1.38 times more into the blood and was retained 1.27 times more in the liver than a USP isolate form [19].

Vitamin B-2, Riboflavin

Naturally exists as riboflavin and various co-enzyme forms in food [10]. In non-foods it is most often synthetically made with 2N acetic acid, is a single form isolate, and is crystalline in structure [1]. Some synthetic riboflavin analogues have weak vitaminic activity [45]. Some natural variations, especially in coenzyme forms, occur in plants, including fungal,

species [45]. An animal study found that Food vitamin B-2 was absorbed 1.49 times more into the blood and was retained 1.92 times more in the liver than a USP isolate form [19]. Various studies suggests that food riboflavin are superior to non-food forms [8,19, 42].

Vitamin 'B-3', Niacinamide

Primarily exists in foods in forms other than niacin [10]. "Niacin is a generic term...the two coenzymes that are the metabolically active forms of niacin (are)...nicotinamide adenine dinucleotide (NAD) and NAD phosphate (NADP)...Only small amounts of free forms of niacin occur in nature. Most of the niacin in food is present as a component of NAD and NADP... nicotinamide is more soluble in water, alcohol, and ether than nicotinic acid...many analogues of niacin have been synthesized, some of which have antivitamin activity " [10]. Niacinamide (also called nicotinamide) is considered to have less potential side-effects than niacin [10]; it also does not seem to cause gastrointestinal upset or hepatotoxicity

that the synthetic time-released niacin can cause [46]. Processing losses for this vitamin are mainly due to water leaching [47]. Isolated, non-food, niacinamide is normally from 3-cyanopyridine and can form crYSTals [1]. This non-food 'niacin' is synthesized from acetaldehyde through several chemical reactions often involving formalydehyde and ammonia [2,48]. Beef, legumes, cereal grains, yeast, and fish are significant natural food sources of vitamin B3 [46]. Animal studies suggest that Food niacinamide is 3.94 times more absorbed in the blood than USP niacinamide and 1.7 times more retained in the liver than a USP isolated niacinamide [19].

Vitamin 'B-5', Pantothenate

Naturally exists in foods as pantothenate [10]. "Pantothenate, usually in the form of CoA, performs multiple roles in cellular metabolism, being central to energy-yielding oxidation of glycolytic products and other metabolites through the mitochondrial tricarboxylic acid cycle...Synthesis of fatty-acids and membrane phospholipids, including regulatory sphingolipids requires pantothenate, and synthesis of the amino acids leucine, arginine, and methionine requires a pantothenate requiring step. CoA is required for synthesis of isoprenoid derivatives, such as cholesterol, steroid hormones, dolichol, vitamin A, vitamin D, and heme A" [10]. "It also appears to be involved in the regulation of gene expression and signal transduction...may have antioxidant and radioprotective properties... It has putative anti-inflammatory, wound healing and antiviral activities...may be helpful in the management of some with rheumatoid arthritis... shown to accelerate wound healing" [33]. "Synthetic D-pantothenate...is available as a calcium or sodium salt" [10], and is sold in forms such as sodium D-pantothenate or calcium D-pantothenate or sometime just listed as pantothenic acid [33]. Other synthetic "multivitamin preparations commonly contain its...alcohol derivative, panthenol" [10]. "Dexopanthenol is a synthetic form which is not found naturally" [33]. USP pantothenic acid is made by condensing isobutyraldehyde with formaldehyde [2]. "Pantothenic acid consists of pantoic acid in amide linkage to beta-alanine", but vitamin B-5 is not found that way in nature [49]. Vitamin B-5 is found in food as pantothenate forms; foods do not naturally contain pantothenic acid [49]. The vegetarian foods which are highest in natural pantothenate are nutritional yeast, brown rice, peanuts, and broccoli [10,32,49]. Specifically, *Saccharomyces cerevisiae* is one of the best natural sources of food pantothenate [10,33]. Calcium pantothenate is a synthetic enantiomer [10] and is a calcium salt [1] and is crystalline [2]. An animal study indicated that Food pantothenate was 1.54% more absorbed into the blood than a USP form [19].

Vitamin B-6

Plants naturally primarily contain vitamin B6 in forms such as 5'0-(beta-D-glycopyransosyl) and other pyridoxines, not pyridoxal forms [10]. Pyridoxine hydrochloride is not naturally found in the body [10], is a crystalline isolate [1], and is generally made from petroleum and hydrochloric acid and processed with formaldehyde [4]. Pyridoxal-5-phosphate is made by combining phosphorus oxychloride and/or adenosine triphosphate with pyridoxal [1]; it becomes a crystalline isolate [1] and bears almost no resemblance to food vitamin B6. At least one synthetic vitamin B-6 analogue has been found to inhibit natural vitamin B-6 action [50,51]. A study of healthy elderly individuals found about 1/3 had marginal vitamin B-6 deficiency [34]. An animal study found that Food vitamin B-6 was absorbed 2.54 times more into the blood and was retained 1.56 times more in the liver than a USP isolate form [19].

Vitamin 'B-9', Folate

Folate was once known as vitamin B-9, as well as vitamin M. Initially food folate was given for people with a pregnancy-related anemia in the form of autolyzed yeast; later a synthetic USP isolate was developed [10]. Pteroylglutamic acid (folic acid), the common pharmacological (USP) form of folate is not found significantly as such in the body [10]. "Folic acid is a synthetic folate form" [52]. Folic acid, such as in most supplements, is not found in food, folates are [15]. Insufficient folate can result in fatigue, depression, confusion, anemia, reduced immune function, loss of intestinal villi, and an increase in infections [11]. Folate deficiency is the most important determinant in high Homocysteine levels [11], and supplemental folate is effective in reducing Homocysteine [53,54]. "The highest concentrations of folate exist in yeast...and brocolli"[10]. "(C)onsumption of more than 266 mcg of synthetic folic acid (PGA) results in absorption of unreduced PGA, which may interfere with folate metabolism for a period of years" [10]. A 2004 paper from the British Medical Journal confirmed what many natural health professionals have known all along: since folic acid is unnatural and the body cannot fully convert large amounts of it into usable folate, this artificial substance can be absorbed and may have unknown negative consequences in the human body [22]--folate supplementation obviously should be in food folate forms and not folic acid. Folic acid is dangerous [24]. An animal study found that Food folate was absorbed 1.07 times more into the blood and was retained 2.13 times more in the liver than a USP isolated folic acid [19].

Vitamin B-12

The naturally active forms are methylcobalamin and deoxyadenosylcobalamin and are found in food [10]. Cyanocobalamin is not a naturally active form [10]; it is an isolate which is crystalline in structure [1]. Initially natural food complex vitamin B12 was given for people with pernicious anemia in the form of raw liver, but due to cost considerations a synthetic USP isolate was developed [7]. According to Dr. Victor Herbert (and others) vitamin B-12 when ingested in its human-active form is non-toxic, yet Dr. Herbert (and others) have warned that "the efficacy and safety of the vitamin B12 analogues created by nutrient-nutrient interaction in vitamin-mineral supplements is unknown" [54]. Some synthetic vitamin B12 analogues seem to be antagonistic to vitamin B12 activity in the body [55,56]. Most synthetic B-12 is made through a fermentation process with the addition of cyanide [4]. An animal study found that Food vitamin B-12 was absorbed 2.56 times more into the blood and was retained 1.59 times more in the liver than a USP isolated form [19].

Vitamin B-x, Vitamin B-8, Vitamin B factors like Choline

PABA was once called vitamin B-x, while inositol was once called vitamin B-8. They and choline are considered to be vitamin B co-factors, as well as lipotropic factors.

In large doses, PABA is "indicated for Peyronie's disease, scleroderma, morphea and linear scleroderma" [11]. The non-food version of PABA is made from coal tar [2]. In addition, there is a non-food potassium salt synthetic form, called aminobenzoate potassium [11]. PABA is found in foods such as kidney, liver, molasses, fungal foods, spinach, and whole grains [57].

The non-food version of inositol is made from phytin processed with sulfuric acid [2]. Inositol is a lipotropic factor, and is also necessary for hair growth; some use it for mood issues. While nutritional yeast is probably the best source of inositol, it is also found in fruits, lecithin, legumes, meats, milk, unrefined molasses, raisins, vegetables, and whole grains [57].

Choline bitartrate and choline chloride, the types most often encountered in allegedly "natural" vitamin supplements, are actually "commercial salts" [11]—they are synthetic forms. Ethylene is involved in the production of one or more of the synthetic forms [2].

Phosphatidyl-choline is the major delivery form of choline, and is naturally found in many foods such as beef liver, egg yolks, and soya [11]. Specially grown nutritional yeast appears to be the best food form for choline supplements.

Vitamin C

Vitamin C naturally occurs in fruits in at least two biologically-active ascorbate forms with bioflavonoids [10]. Non-food, so-called 'natural' ascorbic acid is made by fermenting corn sugar into sorbitol, then hydrogenating it until it turns into sorbose, then acetone (commonly referred to as nail polish remover) is added to break the molecular bonds which creates isolated, crystalline, ascorbic acid. It does not contain both vitamin C forms (nor bioflavonoids), thus is too incomplete to properly be called vitamin C [2]. The patented 'vitamin C' compounds that are touted as less acidic than ascorbic acid also are not food (it is not possible to get a US patent on naturally occurring vitamins as found in food--anytime a health professional hears that some vitamin is patented, that should set off warning signals that it is not real food). An *in vitro* study found that food complex vitamin C has negative ORP (oxidative reductive potential) [27], yet the Merck Index shows that so-called 'natural' ascorbic acid has positive ORP [1] (negative ORP is much better as it helps 'clean up' oxidative damage whereas items with positive ORP do not) [58]. Food complex vitamin C is also 10x less acidic than ascorbic acid.

Some of the many functions vitamin C is involved in include collagen formation, carnitine biosynthesis, neurotransmitter synthesis, enhancement of iron

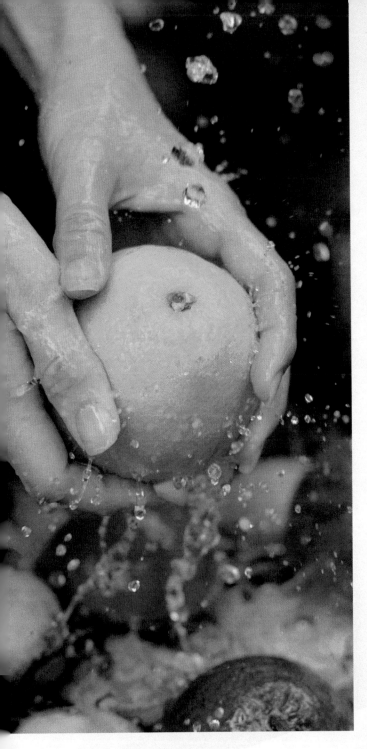

has over 15.6 times the ORAC of isolated ascorbic acid [25] (food complex vitamin C is even higher). Actually, there are doubts that isolated ascorbic acid has any significant antioxidant effects in humans [31]. Food vitamin C is clearly superior for any interested in ORAC.

Although food vitamin C is superior to isolated ascorbic acid [8], at least one mainstream researcher has written, "The bioavailability of vitamin C in food and 'natural form' supplements is not significantly different from that of pure synthetic AA" [10] this is simply not true. As "proof" that particular author cites two papers. The first citation is a study that concludes since serum ascorbic acid levels were at similar levels after various vitamin C containing foods and synthetic ascorbic acid were consumed, that the bioavailability is similar [60]. The conclusions reached seem to ignore that fact that it may be possible that DHAA or other food constituents associated with natural vitamin C may have positive effects other than raising serum ascorbate levels.

The second citation is a study that probably should not have been cited as it never compared vitamin C as complexed in food versus synthetic ascorbic acid (it compared synthetic ascorbic acid to Ester-C which is a commercial blend of synthetic ascorbic acid and select metabolites as well as to synthetic ascorbic acid mixed with some bioflavonoids) [61]. Hence, those who claim that there is no difference really do not have strong scientific proof for their contrary opinion.

A human study found that Food vitamin C was absorbed 1.74 times more into red blood cells than a USP isolated ascorbic acid [62]. Yet another human study found thatl Food vitamin C is absorbed 1.35 times more than plain ascorbic acid [63]. An animal study found that after one month of feeding, Food vitamin C caused a significant reduction of 77%, 66%, and 40% in plasma total cholesterol, LDL + VLDL, and triglycerides respectively and that USP ascorbic acid or bioflavonoids alone were ineffective (though ascorbate did raise HDL); this same study also found that Food vitamin C strongly inhibited atherosclerosis [64]. Spectral Data Services (a nuclear magnetic testing facility) has concluded, regarding Food vitamin C, "the materials have undergone a physical chemical change, they are not a simple mixture" [65]. Various scientific investigations have demonstrated that food vitamin C is superior to isolated ascorbic acid.

absorption, immunocompetence, antioxidant defense, possible anticarcenogenic effects, protection of folate and vitamin E from oxidation, and cholesterol catabolism [1].

One study found that a Food vitamin C had 492 micro moles per gram T.E. (Trolox equivalents) of hydrophilic ORAC (oxygen radical absorbance capacity) [59]—ORAC is essentially a measurement of the ability to quench free radicals (antioxidant ability)—while blueberries (one of the highest ORAC sources [25]) only had 195 micro moles per gram T.E. [59]—thus food vitamin C has 2.52 times the ORAC ability of blueberries. Vitamin C containing food

Vitamin D

The history of synthetic vitamin D is a shocking one. "The first vitamin isolated was a photoproduct from the irradiation of the fungal sterol ergosterol. This vitamin was known as D1...vitamin D obtained from irradiation of ergosterol had little antirachitic activity" [66]--in other words, the first synthetic vitamin D did not act the same as natural vitamin D. "At the time of its identification, it was assumed that the vitamin D made in the skin during exposure to sunlight was vitamin D2", but it was later learned that human skin produced something called vitamin D3 [60]. It was first believed that provitamin D3 was directly converted to vitamin D3, but that was incorrect.

The skin actually contains a substance commonly called provitamin D3; after exposure to sunlight previtamin D3 is produced and it begins to isomerize into vitamin D2 in a process which is temperature dependent, with isomerized vitamin D3 being jettisoned from the plasma membrane into extracellular space. Vitamin D2 was used to fortify milk in the US and Canada for about forty years until it was learned that D3 was the substance which had better antirachitic activity, so D3 has been used for the past twenty-five years [66]. But vitamin D has many benefits which are unrelated to rickets: B and T lymphocytes have been shown to have receptors for vitamin D similar to those found in the intestines, vitamin D seems to affect phagocytosis, and may even have some antiproliferation effect for tumor cells [66].

It has not been proven that any single USP isolated form of vitamin D has all the benefits as natural occurring forms of vitamin D. (Also, since the vitamin D was not particularly stable, manufacturers used to put in 1.5 to 2 times as much of synthetic vitamin D as they claimed on the product labels. This led to neonatal problems and hypercalcemia. [66].) One

older report found that "natural vitamin D is about 100 times more potent in protecting chickens and children from rickets than...irradiated ergosterol" [67], USP vitamin D2. Vegetarian sources of vitamin D include shitake mushrooms and specially grown nutritional yeast.

New vitamin D analogues are still being developed: some which may have greater affects on calcium utilization [69], some even may be helpful for breast cancer [69]--but these really may be pharmacological, and not naturopathic, applications since these analogues are not food. In view of the historical errors in the supplementation with forms of vitamin D, it is reasonable to conclude that additional benefits of natural source vitamin D may be discovered, further distinguishing it from synthetic isolates.

Vitamin D is not an isolate. It exists as a combination of substances (including vitamin D3), with promoting metabolites [10]. Non-food vitamin analogues D1, D2, D3, and D4 are isolates without the promoting metabolites. USP D1 does not have appreciable antirachitic effects [10], is crystalline, and is made with benzene [1]. USP D2 is considered a synthetic form and is made by bombarding ergosterol with electrons [1] and is "recovered by solvent extraction" [2]. USP D3 and D4 are both made through irradiating animal fat [1,10] or through irradiating "the spinal cords and brains of cattle" [2]. Scientists are even developing a 'new' form of vitamin D (which is admitted to be an analogue) which is supposed to be helpful for osteoporosis [70]. Natural vitamins cannot be invented! The fact that some drugs are chemically similar to vitamin D as found in foods, does not make them true vitamins. Food vitamin D has been reported to have at least 10 times the antirachitic effects than one or more isolated USP forms [71].

Vitamin E

Natural vitamin E "as found in foods is [d]-alpha tocopherol, whereas chemical synthesis produces a mixture of eight epimers" [72] (natural vitamin E has recently been renamed to be called RRR-alpha-tocopherol whereas the synthetic has now been renamed to all-rac-alpha-tocopherol, though supplement labels rarely make this clear; on supplement labels d-alpha-tocopherol is generally 'natural', whereas dl-alpha-tocopherol is synthetic [27]).

Natural RRR-alpha-tocopherol has 1.7 - 4.0 times the free radical scavenging strength of the other tocopherols, RRR-alpha tocopherol has 3 times the biological activity of the alpha-tocotrienol form, and synthetic vitamin E simply does not have the same biologic activity of natural vitamin E. Some synthetic forms have only 2% of the biological activity of RRR-alpha-tocopherol [27].

The biologic activity of vitamin E is based on its

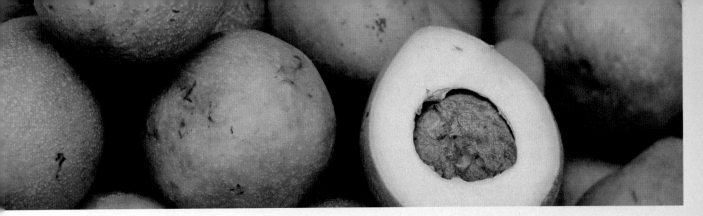

ability to reverse specific vitamin E-deficiency symptoms [27], therefore it is a scientific fact that, overall, synthetic vitamin E has less ability to correct vitamin E deficiencies than food vitamin E. There is an interesting reason for this, which is that the body regulates plasma vitamin E through a specific liver alpha-tocopherol transfer protein, whereas it has no such protein for other vitamin E forms [27]. In other words, the liver produces a protein to handle vitamin E found in food, but not for the synthetic forms. The body retains natural vitamin E 2.7 times better than synthetic forms [32].

Even mainstream researchers teach, "Vitamin E is the exception to the paradigm that synthetic and natural vitamins are the equivalent because their molecular structures are identical...Synthetic vitamin E is produced by commercially coupling trimethylhydroquinone (TMHQ) with isophytol. This chemical reaction produces a difficult-to-separate mixture of eight isomers" [73] (vitamin E, of course, is not the only exception--all nutrients are better if they are Food).

Isolated natural vitamin E has been found to have twice the bioavailability as synthetic vitamin E [74]. The form of vitamin E found in Food has been found to be 2.7 times better retained in the body than a synthetic form [28]—this appears to be because the body attempts to rid itself of synthetic forms as quickly as possible [28]. It is interesting to note that so-called "natural" forms (like succinate) do not even work like Food vitamin E—Even the PDR notes, "d-Alpha-Tocopherol succinate itself has no antioxidant activity" [33], so why would anyone want that for their vitamin E supplement?

Vitamin E is necessary for the optimal development and maintenance of the nervous system as well as skeletal muscle [73]. Vitamin E deficiency can lead to certain anemias, nutritional muscular dYSTrophy, reproductive problems, and hyperlipidemia [72]. Vitamin E has been shown to reduce the risk of various cancers, coronary heart disease, cataract formation, and even the effects of air pollution [27,73]. It also is believed it may slow the aging process and decrease exercise-induced oxidative stress [27,73].

Artificial fats seem to increase the need for vitamin E [75]. Vitamin E content is highest in vegetable oils, also relatively high in avocados (4.31 i.u. each) [76] and rice bran [77]. An animal liver study found that Food vitamin E is 2.6 times more retained than d-alpha tocopheryl acid succinate (which is the 'natural form' once it is isolated from its food complex) [19].

Natural vitamin E as predominantly found in foods is [d]-alpha tocopherol (also called RRR-alpha tocopherol) and is never found as an isolate [10]. The so-called 'natural' forms are most frequently in supplements as isolates, a way they are never found in nature.

Both the chemical form and source of vitamin E may play a role as "chemically synthesized alpha-tocopherol is not identical to the naturally occurring form" [27]. Thus those who claim that a synthetic vitamin, even when it is in the same "chemical form" does not matter are wrong. Also as it is never in the same actual form due to the presence of food constituents, it is never as good as one in a natural, food form. The scientific facts about vitamins demonstrate FOOD vitamins are superior.

Vitamin 'H', Biotin

The only active form found in nature is d-(+) biotin and is usually protein bound [10]. Non-food biotin is normally an isolated, synthesized, crystalline form that is not protein bound [1].

Biotin l-sulfoxide is a lessor used isolated and/or non-food form, involves pimelic acid, is an isolate, and has less than 1% of the vitamin H activity of food biotin [1].

Vitamin K

Vitamin K naturally is found in plants as phylloquinone [10]. Non-food vitamin K3 menadione is now recognized as dangerous and is a synthetic naphthoquinone derivative (naphthalene is a coal tar derivative) [1]. USP K1, also called phylloquinone, is an isolate normally synthesized with p-allylic-nickel [1]. There is another form of vitamin K inadvertently formed during the hydrogenation of oils called dihydro-vitamin K1 [78]; however since the consumption of hydrogenated oils appears to be dangerous [79], it does not seem that this form would be indicated for most humans. Dark leafy vegetables, as well as cabbage [80], appear to be the primary food source of vitamin K [81].

Perhaps it should be mentioned that typical multiple vitamin formulas are dangerous and do not result in optimal health. A study involving 38,772 women in the USA who took synthetic multi-vitamins with ground up rock minerals found that the women died earlier than those who did not take them [82]. Synthetic vitamins are dangerous. Yet, 100% food vitamins and minerals are essential to human health and promote longevity.

Types of Available Vitamins

There are really only two types of vitamins sold: food vitamins and non-food vitamins. Food vitamins will normally state something like "100% Food" on the label. Sometimes the label will also state "No USP nutrients" or "No synthetic nutrients".

Non-food vitamins, however are somewhat less obvious. First of all, no non-food vitamin this researcher has seen says "100% food" on the label and none of them state 'No USP or synthetic nutrients." Thus if none of these expressions are present, it is normally safe to conclude that the vitamins are not from food. If a label states that the product contains USP vitamins or 'pharmaceutical grade' nutrients, then it should be obvious to all naturopathic practitioners that the product is not food.

Also, if a multi-vitamin or a B-complex formula states something to the effect that it "contains no yeast" that is basically a guarantee that it contains synthetic nutrients.

However, just because a company uses the term 'natural' or 'all natural' as a description of its vitamins does not make them, in fact, natural—this is **because the**

US Government has no definition of natural and misapplies the term organic!

Notice the following (bolding in source below):

Some 'natural' products are anything but

Vitamin pills can be synthetically, and legally produced, produced in a lab. Synthetic ingredients are even allowed in multi-vitamins that bear the Department of Agriculture's "Organic" seal...

"Vitamins can be synthetic because, by definition, a vitamin does not have to come from nature," says Fabricant at the FDA. [83]

This is outrageous, and many have been misled. Real vitamins do come from nature and are contained in grown foods. It is terrible, but the reality is that the vast majority of vitamin pills are synthetic.

Also please understand, just because a company may have a reputation for having natural products (like one company that boasts about its farm and many others that use terms like natural), this does not mean

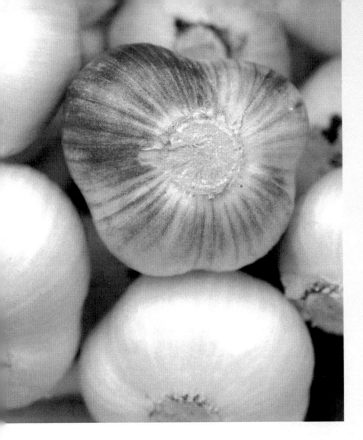

This mixing does not change the chemical form of the vitamin, so it is still a vitamin analogue and not a food vitamin (this differs from food, as true food vitamins are not simple mixture).

Some other companies (that do not use the term 'food-based') mix foods with the vitamin analogue and seem to imply that the vitamin is a food. For example, if a label states something like Vitamin C (Vitamin C, acerola) then it is also normally a synthetic mixed with a food. If the product were a food, it would normally state that the vitamin C was in food or from acerola and not use the term 'vitamin C' twice in a row on the label (many companies mix ascorbic acid with acerola). At least one company that targets health professionals does this.

Many companies use the term 'yeast-free' on their synthetic vitamin labels, apparently implying that yeast should not be used in vitamins. There are a couple of problems with this. The first is that several non-food isolated vitamins are produced by yeast, before they are industrially processed and isolated, thus it is unlikely that any multiple vitamin formula has not been partially made up of yeast, yeast extracts, or yeast by-products [1,2]. The second problem is that nutritional yeast is not the same as brewer's yeast, which is essentially a waste by-product.

its vitamins are not synthetic—carefully check the label for proof that the product is truly 100% food.

Some companies seem to confuse the issue by using the term 'food-based' on their supplement labels. 'Food-based' vitamins are almost always USP vitamins mixed with a small amount of food.

Conclusions

Most vitamins sold are not food--they are synthetically processed petroleum and/or hydrogenated sugar extracts--even if they say "natural" on the label. They are not in the same chemical form or structural form as real vitamins are in foods; thus they are not natural for the human body. True natural food vitamins are superior to synthetic ones [8,16,42]. Food vitamins are functionally superior to non-food vitamins as they tend to be preferentially absorbed and/or retained by the body. Isolated, non-food vitamins, even when not chemically different are only fractionated nutrients.

Studies cited throughout this paper suggest that the bioavailability of food vitamins is better than that of most isolated USP vitamins, that they may have better effects on maintaining aspects of human health beyond traditional vitamin deficiency syndromes, and at least some seem to be preferentially retained by the human body. It is not always clear if these advantages are due to the physiochemical form of the vitamin, with the other food constituents that are naturally found with them, or some combination. Regardless, it seems logical to conclude that for purposes of maintaining normal health, natural vitamins are superior to synthetic ones [8,16,42]. Unlike some synthetic vitamins, no natural vitamin has been found to not perform all of its natural functions.

The truth is that only foods, or supplements composed of 100% foods, can be counted on as not containing non-food vitamin analogues. Natural health advocates are supposed to build health on foods or nutrients contained in foods. That was the standard set for the profession in 1947. That standard—that commitment to real naturopathy—should remain for natural health professionals today.

References

[1] Budvari S, et al editors. The Merck Index: An encyclopedia of Chemicals, Drugs, and Biologicals, 12th ed. Merck Research Laboratories, Whitehouse Station (NJ), 1996

[2] Vitamin-Mineral Manufacturing Guide: Nutrient Empowerment, volume 1. Nutrition Resource, Lakeport (CA), 1986

[3] DeCava JA. The Real Truth About Vitamins and Antioxidants. A Printery, Centerfield (MA), 1997

[4] Hui JH. Encyclopedia of Food Science and Technology. John Wiley, New York, 1992

[5] Gehman JM. From the Office of the President: Pseudo-Group Once Again Misleading the Naturopathic Field. Official Bulletin ANA, January 25, 1948:7-8

[6] Ensminger AH, et al. Food & Nutrition Encyclopedia, 2nxd ed. CRC Press, New York, 1993

[7] Mervyn L. The B Vitamins. Thorsons, Wellingborough (UK), 1981

[8] Thiel R. Natural vitamins may be superior to synthetic ones. Med Hypo 2000 55(6):461-469

[9] Haynes W. Chemical Trade Names and Commercial Synonyms, 2nd ed. Van Nostrand Co., New York, 1955

[10] Shils M, et al, editors. Modern Nutrition in Health & Disease, 9th ed. Williams & Wilkins, Balt.,1999

[11] Gruenwald et al editors. PDR for Herbal Medicines, 2nd ed. Medical Economics Company. Montvale (NJ) 2000

[12] Crook W. The Yeast Connection: A Medical Breakthrough, 3rd ed. Professional Books, Jackson, TN; 1986

[13] Whitney EN, Rolfes S. Understanding Nutrition, 4th ed. West Publishing, New York, 1987

[14] Jenkins DJA, Wolever TMS, and Jenkins AL. Diet Factors Affecting Nutrient Absorption and Metabolism. In Modern Nutrition in Health and Disease, 8th ed. Lea & Febiger, Phil.,1994:583-602

[15] Macrae R, Robson RK, Sadler MJ. Encyclopedia of Food Science and Nutrition. Academic Press, New York, 1993

[16] DeCava, J. The Lee Philosophy-Part II. Nutrition News and Views 2003;7(1):1-6

[17] Jensen B. Chemistry of Man. Bernard Jensen, Escondido (CA), 1983

[18] Lee R. How and Why Synthetic Poisons Sold as Imitations of Natural Foods and Drugs? 1948

[19] Vinson J, Bose P, Lemoine L, Hsiao KH. Bioavailability studies. In Nutrient Availability: Chemical and Biological Aspects. Royal Society of Chemistry, Cambridge (UK) 1989:125-127

[20] Ross A.C. Vitamin A and Carotenoids. In Modern Nutrition in Health and Disease, 10th ed. Lippincott William & Wilkins, Phil, 2005: 351-375

[21] Ha SW. Rabbit study comparing yeast and isolated B vitamins (as described in Murray RP. Natural vs. Synthetic. Mark R. Anderson, 1995:A3). Ann Rev Physiol, 1941;3:259-282

[22] Elvehjem C. Chick study comparing Goldberg diet (as described in Murray RP. Natural vs. Synthetic. Mark R. Anderson, 1995:A4). J Am Diet Assoc, 1940;16(7):654

[23] Lucock M. Is folic acid the ultimate functional food component for disease prevention? BMJ, 2004;328:211-214

[24] Thiel R. Folic Acid is Hazardous to Your Health. What About Food Folate? The Original Internist, 17(2) June 2010, 88-90

[25] Williams D. ORAC values for fruits and vegetables. Alternatives, 1999;7(22):171

[26] Thiel R. Vitamin D, rickets, and mainstream experts. Int J Naturopathy, 2003; 2(1)

[27] Traber MG. Vitamin E. In Modern Nutrition in Health and Disease, 9th ed. Williams & Wilkins, 1999:347-362

[28] Olson R.E. Vitamin K. In Modern Nutrition in Health and Nutrition, 9th ed. Williams & Wilkins, Balt., 1999: 363-380

[29] Thiel R. ORP Study on Durham-produced Food Vitamin C for Food Research LLC. Doctors' Research Inc., Arroyo Grande (CA), February 17, 2006

[30] Fowkes SW. Antioxidants & reduction. Smart Life News, 2000;7(9):6-8

[31] Sebastian J, et al. Vitamin C as an antioxidant: evaluation of its role in disease prevention. J Am Coll Nutr, 2003;22(1):18-35

[32] Traber MG, Elsner A, Brigelius-Flohe R. Synthetic as compared with natural vitamin E is preferentially excreted as alpha-CEHC in human urine: studies using deuterated alpha-tocopherol acetates. FESB Letters, 1998;437:145-148

[33] Hendler S, Rorvik D, editors. PDR for Nutritional Supplements. Medical Economics, Montvale (NJ), 2001

[34] Chu YF, Sun J, Wu X, Liu RH. Antioxidant and antiproliferative activities of common vegetables. J Agric Food Chem. 2002;50(23):6910-6916

[35] Ben-Amotz A, et al. Effect of natural beta-carotene supplementation in children exposed to radiation from the Chernobyl accident. Radiat Environ Biophys 1998;37:187-193

[36] Paolini M, Abdel-Rahman SZ, Sapone A, Pedulli GF, Perocco P, Cantelli-Forti G, Legator MS. Beta-carotene: a cancer chemopreventive agent or a co-carcinogen? Mutat Res. 2003;543(3):195-200

[37] Patrick L. Beta-carotene: the controversy continues. Altern Med Rev. 2000;5(6):530-45

[38] Ben Amotz; van het Hof KH, Gartner C, Wiersma A, Tijburg LB, Westrate JA. Comparison of the bioavailability of natural palm oil carotenoid and synthetic beta-carotene in humans. J Agric Food Chem, 1999;47(4):1582-1586

[39] Bowen HT, Omaye ST. Oxidative changes associated with beta-carotene and alpha-tocopherol enrichment of human low-density lipoproteins. J Am Coll Nutr. 1998;17(2):171-179

[40] Sinatra S. Consumer Alert: Don't Touch this Button, 2003:34-35

[41] Stepp W, Kuhnau J. Schroeder J. The vitamins and their clinical applications (as described in Murray RP. Natural vs. Synthetic. Mark R. Anderson, 1995:A2). Ferdinand Enke, Stuttgart, Germany 1936.

[42] Murray RP. Anderson MR. Natural vs. Synthetic. Mark R. Anderson, 1995:A1-2

[43] Chick H. Rat study comparing fortified white flour to wholegrain flour (as described in Murray RP. Natural vs. Synthetic. Mark R. Anderson, 1995:A3). Lancet, 1940;2:511-512

[44] McCormick DB, Riboflavin. In Modern Nutrition in Health and Disease, 9th ed. William & Wilkins, Balt.,1999:391-399

[45] McCormick DB. Riboflavin. In Modern Nutrition in Health and Disease, 8th ed. Lea & Febiger, Phil.,1994:366-375

[46] Cervantes-Lauren D, McElvaney NG, Moss J. Niacin. In Modern Nutrition in Health and Disease, 9th ed. Williams & Wilkins, Balt.,1999:401-411

[47]Williams AW, Erdman JW. Food processing: nutrition, safety, and quality balances. In Modern Nutrition in Health and Disease, 9th ed. William &

Wilkins, Balt.,1999:1813-1821

[48] Hui JH. Encyclopedia of Food Science and Technology. John Wiley, New York, 1992

[49] Shils M, et al, editors. Modern Nutrition in Health and Disease, 8th ed. Lea & Febiger, Phil.,1994

[50] Nakano H, McMahon LG, Gregory JF. Pyridoxine-5'-beta-glucoside exhibits incomplete bioavailability as a source of vitamin B-6 and partially inhibits the utilization of co-ingested pyridoxine in humans. J Nutr,1997;127(8):1508-1513

[51] Mervyn L. The B Vitamins. Thorsons, Wellingborough (UK), 1981

[52] Verhoef P. Homocysteine metabolism and risk of myocardial infarction: Relation with vitamin B6, B12, and Folate. Am J Epidemiol 1996;143(9):845-859

[53] Brattstrom L. Vitamins as Homocysteine-lowering agents: A mini review. Presentation at The Experimental Biology 1995 AIN Colloquium, April 13, 1995, Atlanta Georgia

[54] Herbert V, Das KC. Folic acid and vitamin B12. In Modern Nutrition in Health and Disease, 8th ed. Lea & Febiger, Phil.,1994:402-425

[55] Ishida A, Kanefusa H, Fujita H, Toraya T. Microbiological activities of nucleotide loop-modified analogues of vitamin B12. Arch Microbiol,1994;161(4):293-299

[56] Tandler B, Krhenbul S, Brass EP. Unusual mitochondria in the hepatocytes of rats treated with a vitamin B12 analogue. Anat Rec,1991;231(1):1-6

[57] Balch JF, Balch PA. Prescription for a Nutritional Healing, 2nd ed. Avery Publishing, Garden City Park (NY), 1997

[58] Thiel RJ. The truth about vitamins in supplements. ANMA Monitor, 2003;6(2):6-14

[59] ORAC Test by Brunswick Laboratories, Wareham (MA), February 2006

[60] Mangels AR, et al. The bioavailability to humans of ascorbic acid from oranges, orange juice and cooked broccoli is similar to that of synthetic ascorbic acid. J Nutr, 1993;123(6):1054-1061

[61] Johnson C, Luo B. Comparison of the absorption and excretion of three commercially available sources of vitamin C. J Am Diet Assoc, 1994;94:779-781

[62] Vinson J. Human supplementation with different forms of vitamin C. University of Scranton, Scranton (PA)

[63] Vinson JA, Bose P. Comparative bioavailabililty of humans to ascorbic acid alone or in a citrus extract. Am J Clin Nutr, 1988;48:601-406

[64] Vinson JA, Hu S, Jung S. A citrus extract plus ascorbic acid decreases lipids, lipid peroxides, lipoprotein oxidative susceptibility, and atherosclerosis in hypercholesterolemic hamsters. J Agric Food Chem, 1998;46:1453-1469

[65] Turner G. Spectral Data Services. Tests conducted Feb. 1993

[66] Holick MF. Vitamin D. In Modern Nutrition in Health and Disease, 9th ed. William & Wilkins, Balt.,1999:329-345

[67] Supplee G, Ansbacher S, Bender R, Flinigan G. Reports on prevention of rickets in chickens and children using natural and USP forms of vitamin D (as described in Murray RP. Natural vs. Synthetic. Mark R. Anderson, 1995:A6). J Biol Chem, 1936;1(107)957

[68] Miyamoto K, Murayama E, Ochi K, Watanabe H, Kubodera N. Synthetic studies of vitamin D analogues. XIV. Synthesis and calcium regulating activity of vitamin D3 analogues bearing a hydroxlkoxy group at the 2 beta-position. Chem Pharm Bull, 1993;41(6):1111-1113

[69] Fioravanti L, Miodini P, Cappelletti V, DiFronzo G. Synthetic analogs of vitamin D3 have inhibitory effects on breast cancer cell lines. Anticancer Res, 1998;18:1703-1708

[70] Research Breakthroughs. USA Weekend, November 15-17, 2002

[71] Thiel R. Vitamin D, rickets, and mainstream experts. Int J Naturopathy, 2003; 2(1):15-19

[72] Farrel PM, Robert RJ. Vitamin E. In Modern Nutrition in Health and Disease, 8th ed. Lea & Febiger, Phil.;1994:326-341

[73] An Overview of Vitamin E Efficacy. VERIS Research Information Service, November 1998

[74] Burton GW, et al. Human plasma and tissue alpha-tocopherol concentrations in response to supplementation with deuterated natural and synthetic vitamin E. Am J Clin Nutr, 1998;67(4):669-684

[75] Schlagheck TG, et al. Olestra's effect on vitamins D and E in humans can be offset by increasing dietary levels of these vitamins. J Nutr,1997;127(8):1666S-1685S

[76] Avocados rise to the top. Nutr Week, 2001;31(24):7

[77] Rice bran, crude. USDA National Nutrient Database for Standard Reference, Release 18, 2005

[78] Booth SL, Pennington JA, Sadowski JA. Dihydro-vitamin K1: primary food sources and estimated dietary intakes in the American diet. Lipids, 1996;31:715-720

[79] Aschero A, Willett WC. Health affects of trans fatty acids. Am J Clin Nutr, 1997;66:1006S-1010S

[80] Cabbage, raw. USDA National Nutrient Database for Standard Reference, Release 18, 2005

[81] Booth SL, Pennington JA, Sadowski JA. Food sources and dietary intakes of vitamin K-1 (phylloquinone) in the American diet: data from the FDA Total Diet Study. J Am Diet Assoc, 1996;96(2):149-154

[82] Mursu J., et al. Dietary Supplements and Mortality Rate in Older WomenThe Iowa Women's Health Study. Arch Intern Med. 2011;171(18):1625-1633

[83] Shortsleeve C. Yet Another Study Confirms Multivitamins Won't Help Your Heart. Men's Health, July 10, 2018

REFLEX NUTRITION ASSESSMENT CHART™

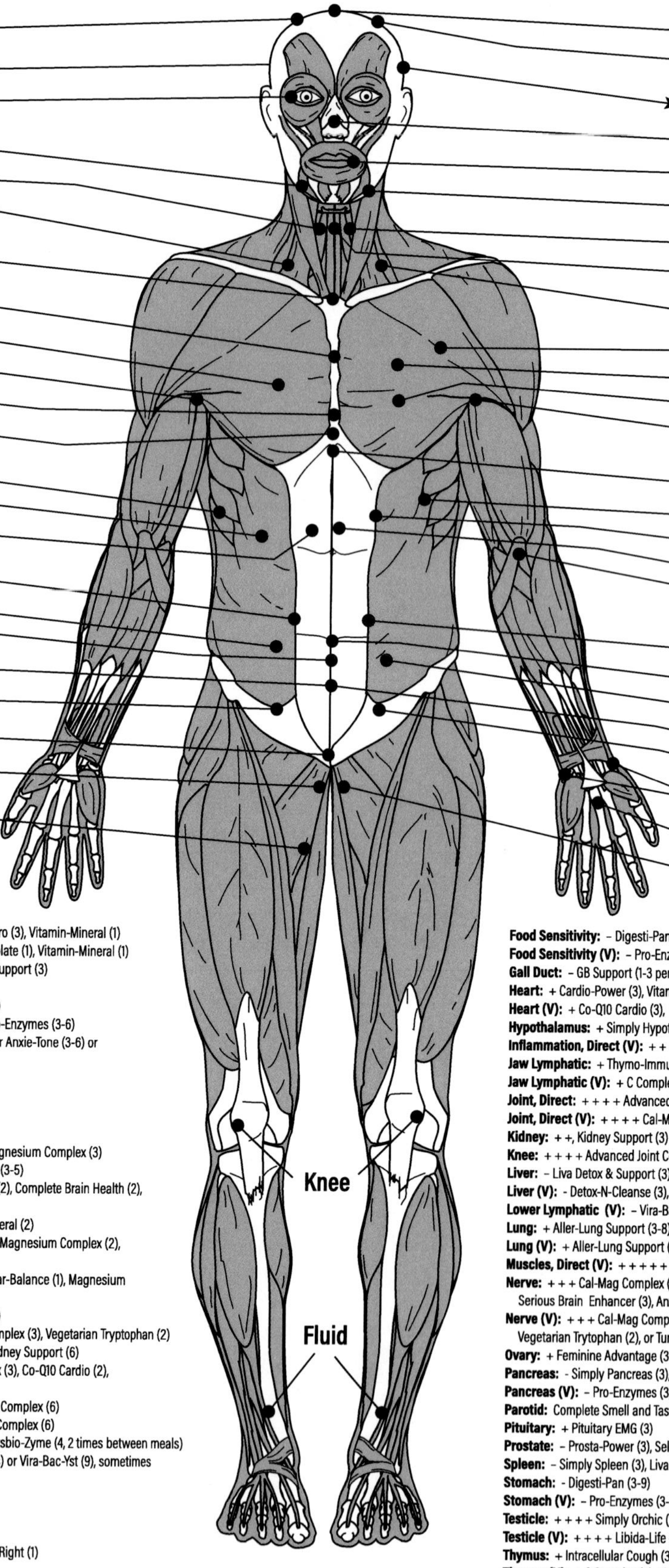

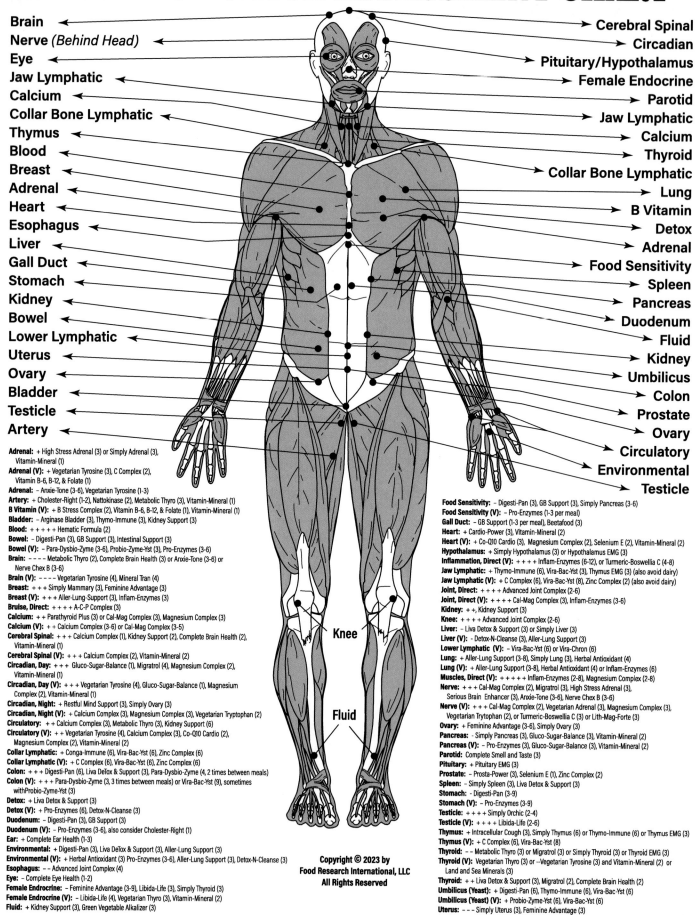

Brain
Nerve *(Behind Head)*
Eye
Jaw Lymphatic
Calcium
Collar Bone Lymphatic
Thymus
Blood
Breast
Adrenal
Heart
Esophagus
Liver
Gall Duct
Stomach
Kidney
Bowel
Lower Lymphatic
Uterus
Ovary
Bladder
Testicle
Artery
Cerebral Spinal
Circadian
Pituitary/Hypothalamus
Female Endocrine
Parotid
Jaw Lymphatic
Calcium
Thyroid
Collar Bone Lymphatic
Lung
B Vitamin
Detox
Adrenal
Food Sensitivity
Spleen
Pancreas
Duodenum
Fluid
Kidney
Umbilicus
Colon
Prostate
Ovary
Circulatory
Environmental
Testicle
Knee
Fluid

Adrenal: + High Stress Adrenal (3) or Simply Adrenal (3), Vitamin-Mineral (1)
Adrenal (V): + Vegetarian Tyrosine (3), C Complex (2), Vitamin B-6, B-12, & Folate (1)
Adrenal: – Anxie-Tone (3-6), Vegetarian Tyrosine (1-3)
Artery: + Cholester-Right (1-2), Nattokinase (2), Metabolic Thyro (3), Vitamin-Mineral (1)
B Vitamin (V): + B Stress Complex (2), Vitamin B-6, B-12, & Folate (1), Vitamin-Mineral (1)
Bladder: – Arginase Bladder (3), Thymo-Immune (3), Kidney Support (3)
Blood: + + + + + + Hematic Formula (2)
Bowel: – Digesti-Pan (3), GB Support (3), Intestinal Support (3)
Bowel (V): – Para-Dysbio-Zyme (3-6), Probio-Zyme-Yst (3), Pro-Enzymes (3-6)
Brain: – – – – Metabolic Thyro (2), Complete Brain Health (3) or Anxie-Tone (3-6) or Nerve Chex B (3-6)
Brain (V): – – – – Vegetarian Tyrosine (4), Mineral Tran (4)
Breast: + + + Simply Mammary (3), Feminine Advantage (3)
Breast (V): + + + Aller-Lung-Support (3), Inflam-Enzymes (3)
Bruise, Direct: + + + + + A-C-P Complex (3)
Calcium: + + Parathyroid Plus (3) or Cal-Mag Complex (3), Magnesium Complex (3)
Calcium (V): + + Calcium Complex (3-6) or Cal-Mag Complex (3-5)
Cerebral Spinal: + + + Calcium Complex (1), Kidney Support (2), Complete Brain Health (2), Vitamin-Mineral (1)
Cerebral Spinal (V): + + + Calcium Complex (2), Vitamin-Mineral (2)
Circadian, Day: + + + Gluco-Sugar-Balance (1), Migratrol (4), Magnesium Complex (2), Vitamin-Mineral (1)
Circadian, Day (V): + + + Vegetarian Tyrosine (4), Gluco-Sugar-Balance (1), Magnesium Complex (2), Vitamin-Mineral (1)
Circadian, Night: + Restful Mind Support (3), Simply Ovary (3)
Circadian, Night (V): + Calcium Complex (3), Magnesium Complex (3), Vegetarian Tryptophan (2)
Circulatory: + + Calcium Complex (3), Metabolic Thyro (3), Kidney Support (6)
Circulatory (V): + + Vegetarian Tyrosine (4), Calcium Complex (3), Co-Q10 Cardio (2), Magnesium Complex (2), Vitamin-Mineral (2)
Collar Lymphatic: + Conga-Immune (6), Vira-Bac-Yst (6), Zinc Complex (6)
Collar Lymphatic (V): + C Complex (6), Vira-Bac-Yst (6), Zinc Complex (6)
Colon: + + + Digesti-Pan (6), Liva DeTox & Support (3), Para-Dysbio-Zyme (4, 2 times between meals)
Colon (V): + + + Para-Dysbio-Zyme (3, 3 times between meals) or Vira-Bac-Yst (9), sometimes withProbio-Zyme-Yst (3)
Detox: + Liva Detox & Support (3)
Detox (V): + Pro-Enzymes (6), Detox-N-Cleanse (3)
Duodenum: – Digesti-Pan (3), GB Support (3)
Duodenum (V): – Pro-Enzymes (3-6), also consider Cholester-Right (1)
Ear: + Complete Ear Health (1-3)
Environmental: + Digesti-Pan (3), Liva DeTox & Support (3), Aller-Lung Support (3)
Environmental (V): + Herbal Antioxidant (3) Pro-Enzymes (3-6), Aller-Lung Support (3), Detox-N-Cleanse (3)
Esophagus: – – Advanced Joint Complex (4)
Eye: – Complete Eye Health (1-2)
Female Endrocrine: – Feminine Advantage (3-9), Libida-Life (3), Simply Thyroid (3)
Female Endrocrine (V): – Libida-Life (4), Vegetarian Thyro (3), Vitamin-Mineral (2)
Fluid: + Kidney Support (3), Green Vegetable Alkalizer (3)

Food Sensitivity: – Digesti-Pan (3), GB Support (3), Simply Pancreas (3-6)
Food Sensitivity (V): – Pro-Enzymes (1-3 per meal)
Gall Duct: – GB Support (1-3 per meal), Beetafood (3)
Heart: + Cardio-Power (3), Vitamin-Mineral (2)
Heart (V): + Co-Q10 Cardio (3), Magnesium Complex (2), Selenium E (2), Vitamin-Mineral (2)
Hypothalamus: + Simply Hypothalamus (3) or Hypothalamus EMG (3)
Inflammation, Direct (V): + + + + Inflam-Enzymes (6-12), or Turmeric-Boswellia C (4-8)
Jaw Lymphatic: + Thymo-Immune (6), Vira-Bac-Yst (3), Thymus EMG (3) (also avoid dairy)
Jaw Lymphatic (V): + C Complex (6), Vira-Bac-Yst (8), Zinc Complex (2) (also avoid dairy)
Joint, Direct: + + + + Advanced Joint Complex (2-6)
Joint, Direct (V): + + + + Cal-Mag Complex (3), Inflam-Enzymes (3-6)
Kidney: + +, Kidney Support (3)
Knee: + + + + Advanced Joint Complex (2-6)
Liver: – Liva Detox & Support (3) or Simply Liver (3)
Liver (V): - Detox-N-Cleanse (3), Aller-Lung Support (3)
Lower Lymphatic (V): – Vira-Bac-Yst (6) or Vira-Chron (6)
Lung: + Aller-Lung Support (3-8), Simply Lung (3), Herbal Antioxidant (4)
Lung (V): + Aller-Lung Support (3-8), Herbal Antioxidant (4) or Inflam-Enzymes (6)
Muscles, Direct (V): + + + + + + Inflam-Enzymes (2-8), Magnesium Complex (2-8)
Nerve: + + + Cal-Mag Complex (2), Migratrol (3), High Stress Adrenal (3), Serious Brain Enhancer (3), Anxie-Tone (3-6), Nerve Chex B (3-6)
Nerve (V): + + + Cal-Mag Complex (2), Vegetarian Adrenal (3), Magnesium Complex (3), Vegetarian Trytophan (2), or Turmeric-Boswellia C (3) or Lith-Mag-Forte (3)
Ovary: + Feminine Advantage (3-6), Simply Ovary (3)
Pancreas: - Simply Pancreas (3), Gluco-Sugar-Balance (3), Vitamin-Mineral (2)
Pancreas (V): – Pro-Enzymes (3), Gluco-Sugar-Balance (3), Vitamin-Mineral (2)
Parotid: Complete Smell and Taste (3)
Pituitary: + Pituitary EMG (3)
Prostate: – Prosta-Power (3), Selenium E (1), Zinc Complex (2)
Spleen: – Simply Spleen (3), Liva Detox & Support (3)
Stomach: - Digesti-Pan (3-9)
Stomach (V): – Pro-Enzymes (3-9)
Testicle: + + + + Simply Orchic (2-4)
Testicle (V): + + + + Libida-Life (2-6)
Thymus: + Intracellular Cough (3), Simply Thymus (6) or Thymo-Immune (6) or Thymus EMG (3)
Thymus (V): + C Complex (6), Vira-Bac-Yst (8)
Thyroid: – – Metabolic Thyro (3) or Migratrol (3) or Simply Thyroid (3) or Thyroid EMG (3)
Thyroid (V): Vegetarian Thyro (3) or --Vegetarian Tyrosine (3) and Vitamin-Mineral (2) or Land and Sea Minerals (3)
Thyroid: + + Liva Detox & Support (3), Migratrol (2), Complete Brain Health (2)
Umbilicus (Yeast): + Digesti-Pan (6), Thymo-Immune (6), Vira-Bac-Yst (6)
Umbilicus (Yeast) (V): + Probio-Zyme-Yst (6), Vira-Bac-Yst (6)
Uterus: – – – Simply Uterus (3), Feminine Advantage (3)

NOTE: "—" refers to ulnar and "+" refers to palmar reflexes. The term DIRECT refers to a position where a problem is apparently existing and NOT a reflex show on this chart.

The Truth About Minerals in Nutritional Supplements

ABSTRACT: *Even though natural health professionals agree that humans should not try to consume industrial chemicals, most seem to overlook this fact when mineral supplementation is involved. And even though many people interested in natural health take minerals, the truth is that nearly all the minerals taken are "natural" for nothing except plants and/or industrial chemicals. While plants are designed to ingest and break-down minerals, humans are not. The truth about nearly all minerals in supplements is that they are really industrial chemicals made from processing rocks with one or more acids. The consumption of this "other half" of the mineral compound is not only unnatural, it can lead to toxicity concerns. Humans were designed to eat food and to get their minerals from foods. Foods DO NOT naturally contain minerals bound to substances such as picolinic acid, carbonates, oxides, phosphates, etc. When supplementation is indicated, only supplements made from 100% food should be considered for supporting optimal health.*

In a nutritional context, minerals are certain elements, such as iron and phosphorus that are essential for the physiology of living organisms to exist.

When it comes to nutrition, plants and humans differ: "a typical plant makes its own food from raw materials... A typical animal eats its food" [1]. For plants, these raw materials include soil-based inorganic mineral salts [2]. Soil-based mineral salts can be depleted through synthetic fertilizers, herbicides, pesticides, as well as repeatedly growing crops on the same soil [3,4].

Plants, with the aid of enzymes and soil-based microorganisms, can take in from soil the mineral salts that they have an affinity for through their roots or hyphae [4]. After various metabolic processes, when these minerals no longer exist as salts, they become complexed with various carbohydrates, lipids, and proteins present in the plant as part of the living organism [5]. Thus for nutrition, humans eat plants and/or animals that eat plants, whereas plants can obtain their nutrients from the soil [4]. This process is commonly referred to as the "food chain" [5].

Unfortunately most mineral supplements contain minerals in the form referred to as 'mineral salts'. Even though mineral salts are often called "natural", they are rocks (e.g. calcium carbonate exists as the rock commonly known as limestone) or they are chemically produced in accordance with the United States Pharmacopoeia (USP). Mineral salts are natural food for plants, they are not a natural food for humans--humans do not have roots or hyphae!

Dietary Guideline number 18 of the Weston A. Price Foundation, an organization devoted to consuming real foods, is: "Use only natural, food-based supplements" [6]. One of the standards of naturopathy agreed to in 1947 was, "Naturopathy does not make use of synthetic or inorganic vitamins or minerals" [7]. Why would naturopaths have mentioned minerals since they are 'natural'? Because even back then, most naturopaths knew that the inorganic minerals being placed into supplements were often simply industrial rocks and not foods. Little has changed in over seven decades since. This paper documents the availability, sources, and some of the chemical differences between minerals found in foods and the industrially processed mineral salts that are found in most 'natural' mineral supplements.

Absorption

Mineral absorption is affected by many factors including the chemical form, structural form, existence or lack of protein chaperones, health, dietary factors, and even medications.

"Absorptive efficiency for many minerals is governed by homeostatic feedback regulation. When the body is in a depleted state, the intestine upregulates absorption of the nutrient. At the biochemical level, this regulation must be expressed by the control of intraluminal binding lignans, cell-surface receptors, intracellular carrier proteins, intracellular storage proteins, or the energetics of the transmembrane transport...In general mineral bioavailability decreases because of many drugs, decreases with age, and in the presence of malnutrition, is associated with poorer integrity of the small intestine. Therefore, older individuals who are often taking numerous medications and who are eating more poorly than young people are at greater risk of mineral deficiencies" [8].

Chemical Differences

The basic difference between minerals found in foods and those found in industrial mineral salts is chemical.

"The chemical form of a mineral is an important factor in its absorption and bioavailability...there is evidence that the form in which minerals are ingested affects absorption. For example, particle size, surface area, and solubility of a substance affects its dilution rate...In many solid foods, elements are not free, but firmly bound in the food matrix" [8].

This, of course, is not true of most minerals in supplements as they are normally industrially processed inorganic rocks (mineral salts) hence they are void of the factors found in a food matrix. Only 100% food minerals have minerals attached in a food matrix.

Minerals are normally found in food; and in the body they are attached with some peptide [9,10]. When humans eat plants or animals they are consuming minerals in those forms. Humans are not supposed to directly consume soil components [1]. With the exception of sodium chloride (common table salt), humans do not normally in any significant quantity consume minerals in the chemical forms known as mineral salts. When they do, it is considered to be a disorder called 'geophagia' or 'pica' [11,12].

It is a fact that mineral salts are often called "natural", but they are not food minerals. Mineral salts are normally inorganic molecular compounds that look like rocks [13]. Mineral salts are a compound containing a mineral element, which is the mineral normally listed on a supplement label, and some other substance it is chemically bound to. Mineral salts are either rocks (e.g. calcium carbonate exists as the rock commonly known as limestone) or they are rocks that are chemically-altered.

Mineral salts are natural food for plants which can chemically change and detoxify them [14]. They are not a natural food for humans, although some people do consider crushed bones and naturally-calcified sea algae, etc. as food. Minerals bound in mineral salts simply are not treated the same way in the body as are minerals found in food.

Minerals vs. Industrial Chemicals

The following list describes what many mineral salts/chelates used in supplements actually are and what they are used for when not in supplements:

Boric acid is the rock known as sassolite. It is used in weatherproofing wood, fireproofing fabrics, and as an insecticide [15].

Calcium ascorbate is calcium carbonate processed with ascorbic acid and acetone. It is a manufactured product used in 'non-food' supplements [15].

Calcium carbonate is the rock known as limestone or chalk. It is used in the manufacture of paint, rubber, plastics, ceramics, putty, polishes, insecticides, and inks. It is also used in fillers for adhesives, matches, pencils, crayons, linoleum, insulating compounds, and welding rods [15].

Calcium chloride is calcium carbonate and chlorine and is the byproduct of the Solvay ammonia-soda process. It is used for antifreeze, refrigeration, fire extinguisher fluids, and to preserve wood and stone. Other uses include cement, coagulant in rubber manufacturing, controlling dust on unpaved roads, freezeproofing of coal, and increasing traction in tires [15].

Calcium citrate is calcium carbonate processed with lactic and citric acids. It is used to alter the baking properties of flour [15].

Calcium gluconate is calcium carbonate processed with gluconic acid, which is used in cleaning compounds. It is used in sewage purification and to prevent coffee powders from caking [15].

Calcium glycerophosphate is calcium carbonate processed with dl-alpha-glycerophosphates. It is used in dentifrices, baking powder, and as a food stabilizer [15].

Calcium hydroxyapatite is crushed bone and bone marrow. It is used as a fertilizer [16].

Calcium iodide is calcium carbonate processed with iodine. It is an expectorant [15].

Calcium lactate is calcium carbonate processed with lactic acid. It is used as a dentifrice and as a preservative [15].

Calcium oxide is basically burnt calcium carbonate. It is used in bricks, plaster, mortar, stucco, and other building materials. It is also used in insecticides and fungicides [15].

Calcium phosphate, tribasic is the rock known as oxydapatit or bone ash. It is used in the manufacture of fertilizers, milk-glass, polishing powders, porcelain, pottery, and enamels [15].

Calcium stearate is an octodecanoic calcium salt and can be extracted from animal fat. It is used for waterproofing fabrics and in the production of cement, stucco, and explosives [15].

Chromium chloride is a preparation of hexahydrates. It is used as a corrosion inhibitor and waterproofing agent [15].

Chromium picolinate is chromium III processed with picolinic acid. Picolinic acid is used in herbicides [17].

Copper aspartate is made "from the reaction between cupric carbonate and aspartic acid (from chemical synthesis)" [18]. It is a manufactured product used in 'non-food' supplements [18].

Copper (cupric) carbonate is the rock known as malachite. It is used as a paint and varnish pigment, plus as a seed fungicide [15].

Copper gluconate is copper carbonate processed with gluconic acid. It is used as a deodorant [19].

Copper (cupric) glycinate is a copper salt processed with glycine. It is used in photometric analysis for copper [15].

Copper sulfate is copper combined with sulfuric acid. It is used as a drain cleaner and to induce vomiting; it is considered as hazardous heavy metal by the City of Lubbock, Texas that "can contaminate our water supply" [20].

Dicalcium phosphate is the rock known as monetite, but can be made from calcium chloride and sodium phosphate. It is used in 'non-food' supplements [18].

Ferric pyrophosphate is an iron rock processed with pyrophosphoric acid. It is used in fireproofing and in pigments [15].

Ferrous lactate is a preparation from isotonic solutions. It is used in 'non-food' supplements [15].

Ferrous sulfate is the rock known as melanterite. It is used as a fertilizer, wood preservative, weed-killer, and pesticide [15].

Magnesium carbonate is the rock known as magnesite. It is used as an antacid, laxative, and cathartic [15].

Magnesium chloride is magnesium ammonium chloride processed with hydrochloric acid. It fireproofs wood, carbonizes wool, and is used as a glue additive and cement ingredient [15].

Magnesium citrate is magnesium carbonate processed with acids. It is used as a cathartic [15].

Magnesium glycinate is a magnesium salt processed with glycine. It is used in 'non-food' supplements.

Magnesium oxide is normally burnt magnesium carbonate. It is used as an antacid and laxative [15].

Manganese carbonate is the rock known as rhodochrosite. It is used as a whitener and to dry varnish [15].

Manganese gluconate is manganese carbonate or dioxide processed with gluconic acid. It is a manufactured item used in 'non-food' supplements [15].

Manganese sulfate is made "from the reaction between manganese oxide and sulfuric acid" [18]. It is used in dyeing and varnish production [15].

Molybdenum ascorbate is molybdenite processed with ascorbic acid and acetone. It is a manufactured item used in 'non-food' supplements [21].

Molybdenum disulfide is the rock known as molybdenite. It is used as a lubricant, additive and hydrogenation Catalyst [15].

Potassium chloride is a crystalline substance consisting of potassium and chlorine. It is used in photography [15].

Potassium iodide is made from HI and KHC03 by melting in dry hydrogen and undergoing electrolysis. It is used to make photographic emulsions and as an expectorant [15].

Potassium sulfate appears to be prepared from the elements in liquid ammonia. It is used as a fertilizer and to make glass [15].

Selenium oxide is made by burning selenium in oxygen or by oxidizing selenium with nitric acid. It is used as a reagent for alkaloids or as an oxidizing agent [15].

Seleniomethionine is a selenium analog of methionine. It is used as a radioactive imaging agent [15].

Silicon dioxide is the rock known as agate. It is used to manufacture glass, abrasives, ceramics, enamels, and as a defoaming agent [15].

Vanadyl sulfate is a blue crystal powder known as vanadium oxysulfate. It is used as a dihydrate in dyeing and printing textiles, to make glass, and to add blue and green glazes to pottery [15].

Zinc acetate is made from zinc nitrate and acetic anhydride. It is used to induce vomiting [15].

Zinc carbonate is the rock known as smithsonite or zincspar. It is used to manufacture rubber [15].

Zinc chloride is a combination of zinc and chlorine. It is used as an embalming material [15].

Zinc citrate is smithsonite processed with citric acid. It is used in the manufacture of some toothpaste [15].

Zinc gluconate is a zinc rock processed with gluconic acid. Gluconic acid is used in many cleaning compounds [15].

Zinc lactate is smithsonite processed with lactic acid. Lactic acid is used as a solvent [15].

Zinc monomethionine is a zinc salt with methionine. It is used as a 'non-food' supplement.

Zinc orotate is a zinc rock processed with orotic acid. Orotic acid is a uricosuric (promotes uric acid excretion) [15].

Zinc oxide is the rock known as zincite. It is used as a pigment for white paint and as part of quick-drying cement [15].

Zinc phosphate is the rock known as hopeite. It is used in dental cements [15].

Zinc picolinate is a zinc rock processed with picolinic acid. Picolinic acid is used in herbicides [17].

Zinc sulfate can be a rock processed with sulfuric acid. It is used as a corrosive in calico-printing and to preserve wood [15].

There is a relatively easy way to tell if minerals are industrial chemicals. Whenever there are two-words on a label describing a mineral, it is a logical to conclude that the substance is an industrial mineral product and not 100% food. The exception is chromium GTF (the GTF stands for glucose tolerance factor) which is food if it is from nutritional yeast [18].

Chelated Minerals

Chelated minerals are generally crushed industrial rocks that are processed with one or more acids.

Probably the biggest difference in minerals now compared to 1947 is that some companies have decided to industrially produce versions of minerals attached to peptides. Essentially they take a rock or industrial mineral salt, chemically alter it, and attempt to attach it to the mineral. This results in a mineral that is different from normal mineral salts, but does not turn the substance into a food. Examples of this include the various mineral ascorbates, picolinates, aspartates, glycinates, and chelates. It must be understood that since there is not a universally accepted definition of the term 'chelate', when this term is used on a label, one generally does not know if the chelate is amino-acid based or some type of industrial acid.

While it is true that humans can, and do, utilize minerals from USP mineral salts or chelated minerals, this is not as safe (or even normally as effective) as consuming them from foods (or in the case of real food supplements, food concentrates).

Non-Food Attachments, Including Some "Chelates," Are Not Desirable

Is it wise to consume non-food minerals?

Dr. Bernard Jensen, an early 20th century advocate of food-based nutrition, once wrote, "When we take out from foods some certain salt, we are likely to alter the chemicals in those foods. When extracted from food, that certain chemical salt is extracted, may even become a poison. Potash by itself is a poison, whether it comes from a food or from the drugstore. This is also the case with phosphorus. You thereby overtax your system, and your functions must work harder in order to throw off those inorganic salts or poisons introduced... The chemical elements that build our body must be in biochemical, life-producing form. They must come to us as food, magnetically, electrically alive, grown from the dust of the earth... When we are lacking any element at all, we are lacking more than one element. There is no one who ever lacked just one element. We don't have a food that contains only one element, such as a carrot entirely of calcium or sprouts totally made of silicon" [22].

It should be noted that the addition of "citric acid and picolinic acid do not appear to enhance zinc absorption" [23]. Chromium picolinate is a human-made substance, created by Gary Evans [24]; it is not a natural food. Picolinic acid is used in herbicides [17]; furthermore "picolinic acid is an excretory or waste product. It is not metabolized by or useful to the body" [25]. Scientists report, "some research groups recently suggested that chromium (III) picolinate produces significantly more oxidative stress and potential DNA damage than other chromium supplements" [26].

Concerns are being raised from various sources about the implications of intentional ingestion of inorganic substances in supplements by human beings [22,25,26]. These substances are not natural for humans to consume and a long period of consumption may cause some type of toxic accumulation [22,25,26]. Yet, many people supposedly interested in natural health are daily consuming various carbonates, gluconates, oxides, picolinates, phosphates, sulfates and other rock components that were not intended to be ingested that way. Since there are many possible negative implications associated with "the other half" of these non-food minerals [25], people truly interested in their health would be much better off consuming foods that are high in minerals or supplements made from those foods.

Jay Patrick claims to have originally developed procedures to manufacture all seven of the mineral ascorbates [21]; thus it would seem highly inappropriate to call supplements with ascorbate attached minerals 'food'.

Actually, it does not appear that any of the minerals marketed as 'chelated' are food concentrates, though there are foods which contain naturally chelated minerals, but these are normally marketed as food minerals. Even though there are some theoretical advantages to industrially-produced mineral 'chelates' as compared to inorganic mineral salts, these chelates are not natural food.

More on Bioavailability

It is well known among nutrition researchers that most essential minerals are not well absorbed; for some minerals, absorption is less than 1% [27]. "Bioavailability of orally administered vitamins, minerals, and trace elements is subject to a complex set of influences...In nutrition science the term 'bioavailability' encompasses the sum of impacts that may reduce or foster the metabolic utilization of a nutrient" [28]. Research demonstrates that the bioavailability and/or effectiveness of mineral containing foods is greater than that of isolated inorganic mineral salts or mineral chelates [e.g. 28-52]. These studies have concluded that natural food minerals may be better absorbed, utilized, and/or retained than mineral salts.

Furthermore, minerals used in most supplements do not contain protein chaperones or other food factors needed for absorption into the cell. In 1999, the Nobel Prize for medicine was awarded to Guenter Blobel who discovered that minerals need protein chaperones to be absorbed into cellular receptors. When mineral salts without protein chaperones are consumed, "It is after digestion when other mineral forms {mineral salts} have their mineral cleaved from their carriers. In this situation, these minerals become charged ions, and their absorbability is in jeopardy. These charged free minerals are known to block the absorption of one another, or to combine with other dietary factors to form compounds that are unabsorbable" [53]. The body must discard the residual chemicals.

Foods used in supplements that commonly provide significant quantities of essential minerals include dulse, horsetail herb, kelp, nutritional yeast, rice bran, and water thyme. These types of foods have been shown to contain not only minerals in natural food forms, but also important protein chaperones such as ATX1 and ceruplasmin [54,55]. Industrial mineral salts do not contain the protein chaperones or other food factors needed for proper mineral absorption. Furthermore, some foods also contain factors which reduce the probability of certain minerals to be toxic to the body [32,33,55]; industrial mineral salts and chelates are simply not that complete.

Quantitative and Qualitative Differences

There are quantitative and qualitative differences in food vs. non-food minerals. Table 1 lists some of them by mineral.

Table 1. Quantitative and Qualitative Differences

Food Mineral	Compared to Mineral Salt/Chelate
Calcium	Up to 8.79 times more absorbed into the blood [47] and 7 times as effective in raising serum ionic calcium levels [30].
Chromium	Up to 25 times more bioavailable [31].
Copper	85% more absorbed [45]; also contains substances that reduce potential toxicity [32,46].
Iron	Safer, non-constipating, 77% more absorbed [33, 34, 45].
Magnesium	Up to 2.20 times better absorbed [52] and retained [35].
Manganese	Better absorbed and retained [45,46] and not as likely to contribute to toxicity as mined forms [36,56].
Molybdenum	Up 6.28 times better absorbed into the blood and 16.49 times better retained [45].
Phosphorus	Less likely to cause diarrhea or electrolyte disorders [37].
Selenium	17.6 times the antioxidant effect [46], 123.01 times more effective in preventing nonenzymatic protein glycation [17], and 2.26 times better retained [29,38,44].
Vanadium	Safer and 50% more effective [39].
Zinc	Up to 6.46 times better absorbed [45,46,51], better form [40,41].

Foods, almost by definition, are not toxic, and as mentioned earlier, can have protective factors to prevent certain potential mineral toxicities, such as those sometimes associated with copper, iron, manganese, or other minerals [32,33,55,56].

Information by Individual Mineral

Some differences between food complexed minerals and mineral salts have been documented by published research and are shown by individual mineral below:

Boron

"Boron complexes with organic compounds containing hydroxyl groups" [9], which is how it is found in foods. Boron affects macromineral and steroidal hormone metabolism; without sufficient boron bone composition, strength, and structure weaken [9].

Calcium

"The amount of calcium absorbed depends on its interaction with other dietary constituents...The absorbability of calcium is mainly determined by the presence of other food constituents" [56]. This is one of the reasons why isolated calcium mineral salts (such as calcium carbonate) are not absorbed as well as calcium found in natural food complexes [56,57]. "Calcium carbonate, an antacid, counteracts not only the absorption of calcium, but also the absorption of iron" [11] (though its calcium absorption appears to be better with food [58]). At least one researcher has concluded that commonly used mineral salts such as calcium lactate and calcium gluconate primarily succeed in creating high blood calcium levels (hypercalcemia) instead of alleviating symptoms of low tissue calcium [59]. "Calcium has a structural role in bones and teeth" as well as in some enzymes involved with blood clotting [48]. Calcium can affect mood and blood pressure [57,60]. Clinical reports consistently confirm that dietary/food calciums [5-8] are important in the management of blood pressure. This does not appear to be the case with isolated calcium salts (the results appear inconsistent [30,61-63]).

One study found that calcium in Food raised serum ionic calcium levels from 1.08 to 1.15 mmoles, but that serum ionic calcium levels were not raised with calcium carbonate [30]. Serum calcium levels affect blood pressure [60,64]. Since low bone mass is somewhat inversely correlated with high levels of diastolic blood pressure [64], this suggests that calcium from Food may be superior when hypertension issues are present. Calcium is important for optimal health as calcium deficiencies can contribute to osteoporosis, muscle (especially the legs) cramps, insomnia, mood/behavioral/nerve problems, hypertension, kidney stones, and colon cancer [61,65,66]. It appears that overdose of calcium can only occur when taking mineral salt forms of calcium supplement as opposed to food [66]. A human study found that Natural Food Complex calcium is 8.79 times more bioavailable than calcium carbonate (which is the most common form found in supplements) and 2.97 times more than calcium gluconate [47]. This same study found that Food calcium "produced no undesirable side effects and was the most suitable form of calcium for long-term supplementation" [47].

Chromium, GTF

"The biologically active form of chromium, sometimes called glucose tolerance factor or GTF, has been proposed to be a complex of chromium, nicotinic acid, and possibly the amino acids glycine, cysteine, and glutamic acid. Many attempts have been made to isolate or synthesize the glucose tolerance factor; none have been successful" [67]. Chromium is not naturally found in the body in the commonly supplemented forms such as chromium picolinate or chromium chelate. "Chromium is generally accepted as an essential nutrient that potentiates insulin action, and thus influences carbohydrate, lipid, and protein metabolism" [67]. Research suggests that there is much less likelihood of toxicity from natural food complex chromium than from forms such as chromium picolinate [26]. Only 1% or less of inorganic chromium is absorbed vs.10-25% of chromium GTF [31]. One small study found that Food chromium GTF reduced blood glucose levels by 16.8% versus 6.0% for inorganic chromium [48], thus it was 2.80 times more effective. One study found that Food chromium benefited certain diabetics by improving blood glucose control, lowering serum lipids, and decreasing the risk of coronary heart disease [49]. Chromium GTF only comes from nutritional yeast [58].

Copper

In the human body, in addition to various plasma-bound coppers, "at least one copper peptide complex" has been isolated [60]. Copper is predominantly found in Food nutrients in a copper peptide complex (such as Cu/Zn superoxide-dismutase). Copper is not naturally found in the body in the form of copper gluconate or copper sulfate. "Anemia, neutropenia, and osteoporosis are observed with copper deficiency." Copper is involved in connective tissue, iron metabolism, the central nervous system, melanin pigment, thermal regulation,

cholesterol metabolism, immune function, and cardiac function [60]. Copper in foods like nutritional yeast contains protective factors that reduce the possibility of toxicity issues [32,46]. A human study found that Food copper was 1.44 times more absorbed into the blood than copper sulfate and 1.43 times more than copper gluconate [45]. Animal studies showed similar results, plus concluded that Food copper was retained in the liver 1.85 times more than copper gluconate and 1.42 times more than copper sulfate [45].

Iron

Most researchers acknowledge that organic iron is better absorbed than inorganic iron [71]. The body has different mechanisms for the absorption of iron depending upon its form [72]. Iron in foods is found in an organic form. Iron is required for growth and hemoglobin formation; inadequate amounts can lead to "weakness, fatigue, pallor, dyspnea on exertion, palpitation, and a sense of being overly tired" [72].

Iron in food is safer, less-constipating (actually it is non-constipating), and better absorbed than non-food forms [33,34]. An animal study found that Food iron was absorbed into the blood 1.01 times more than ferrous sulfate and 1.77 times more than amino acid chelated iron and was retained in the liver 1.21 times more than ferrous sulfate and 1.68 times more than amino acid chelated iron [45,46].

Magnesium

"The percentage of absorption of ingested magnesium is influenced by its dietary concentration and by the presence of inhibiting or promoting dietary components [73]. There are no promoting dietary components in inorganic isolated magnesium salts. "Magnesium is involved in many enzymatic steps in which components of food are metabolized and new products are formed": it is involved in over 300 such reactions [6]. Clinical deficiency of magnesium

can results in "depressed tendon reflexes, muscle fasciculations, tremor, muscle spasm, personality changes, anorexia, nausea, and vomiting" [73]. Magnesium in foods is better absorbed and retained than magnesium from inorganic mineral salts [35]. A human study found that Natural Food Complex magnesium was 2.20 times more absorbed into blood than magnesium oxide and 1.60 times more than amino acid chelated magnesium [52].

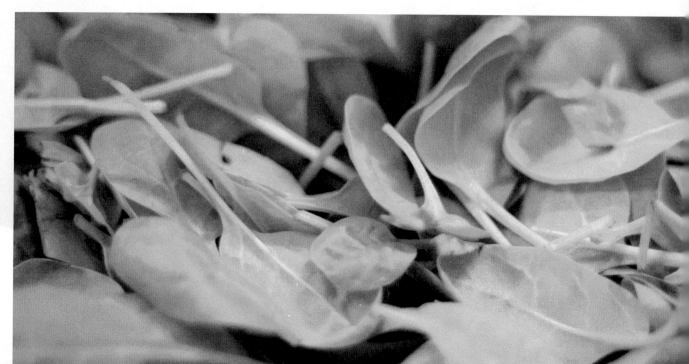

Manganese

In the body, absorbed manganese complexes with various peptides [9]. Manganese is predominantly found in foods in a manganese peptide complex (such as Mn superoxide-dismutase). It is not found in the body in forms like manganese sulfate. Manganese deficiency can cause "impaired growth, skeletal abnormalities, disturbed or depressed reproductive function, ataxia of the newborn, and defects in lipid and carbohydrate metabolism" [9].

It can also affect skin, hair, nails, and problems with calcium metabolism [9]. Manganese in foods is safer and much less likely to cause any toxicity compared to mined forms [36,56]. An animal study found that Natural Food Complex manganese was absorbed 1.56 times more into the blood and was retained 1.63 times more in the liver than manganese sulfate [45,46].

Molybdenum

Molybdenum...in foods...is readily absorbed" [9].

"Molydenum in {nearly all} nutritional supplements is in the form of either sodium molybdate or ammonium molybdate. Molybdenum in food is principally in the form of molydenum cofactors" [67]. "Molybdenum functions as an enzyme cofactor", thus "detoxifies

various pyrimidines, purines, pteridines, and related compounds" [9]; it may also affect growth and reproduction [9]. An animal study found that Food molybdenum was absorbed 6.28 times more into the blood and was retained 16.49 times more in the liver than ammonium molybdate and 10.27 times more than molybdenum amino acid chelate [45].

Phosphorus

Phosphorus is found in plants [11]. Phosphorus salts can cause diarrhea and other problems [37]—problems that do not happen with phosphorus in

foods. Phosphorus works with calcium to produce strong bones [57].

Potassium

Potassium is found in plants [11]. Potassium is the leading intracellular electrolyte and is necessary for electrolyte balance, stimulating aldersterone for the

adrenal glands, and blood pressure regulation [11]. Dr. Bernard Jensen seemed to believe potassium is only safe in its natural food complex form [22].

Selenium

"The predominant form of selenium in animal tissues is selenocysteine" [74]. That is how it is predominantly found in certain foods. One study found that diets naturally high in selenium (daily consumption as high as 724mcg) produced no signs or symptoms of selenium overexposure while another found that exceedingly high consumption of selenium salts could induce selenium poisoning [74]. Selenium seems to support thyroid hormone production, function as part of many enzymes, and have antioxidant effects [74]. Larry Clark, Ph.D. and others have found that selenium in yeast appears to reduce risk of certain cancers [75]. Julian Whitaker, M.D. reports, "The best absorbed form of selenium, and the one used by Dr. Clark's research, is high-selenium yeast" [75]. A study using 247 mcg/day

of high-selenium yeast found that plasma selenium levels were 2-fold higher than baseline values after 3 and 9 months and returned to 136% of baseline after 12 months, whereas there was a 32% increase in blood glutathione levels also seen after 9 months [29]. Food selenium is about twice as well retained as non-food forms [29,38]. Research suggests that Food selenium is 2.26 times more retained in the liver and 1.22 times more absorbed in the blood than sodium selenite [44]. An *in vitro* study found that Food selenium had 17.6 times the antioxidant effect than did selenomethionine [44]. One study found that Food selenium was 123.01 times more effective than sodium selenite in preventing nonenzymatic glycation in diabetics [50].

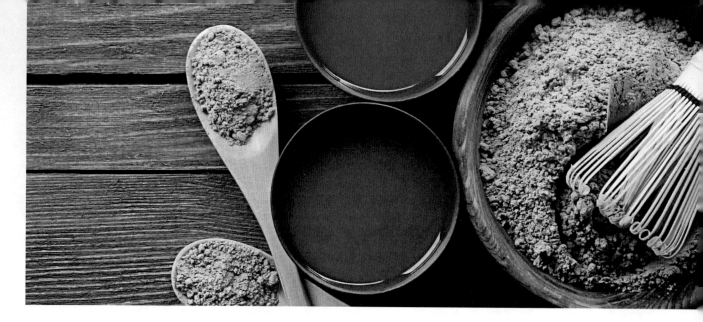

Silicon

"In animals, silicon is found both free and bound" [9]. Silicon absorption is quite dependent upon the form [9]. Silicon is involved in bone calcification and connective tissue formation [9]. It is also needed for healthy hair and skin [51]. Silicon is found in foods in an organic form.

Trace Minerals

Trace minerals, including "ultra trace minerals" are necessary for the proper functioning of human health [9,51]. There are many in the human body, some of which are known to be essential and others of which are under investigation for "essentialness." Sea vegetables and certain yeasts are a good source of trace minerals [11,31,61].

Vanadium

"Vanadate forms compounds with other biological substances" [9]. "Vanadium has been postulated to play a role in the regulation of (NaK)-ATPase, phosphoryl transferase enzymes, adenylate cyclase, and protein kinases; as an enzyme cofactor in the form of vanadyl and in hormone, glucose, lipid, and tooth metabolism" [9]. Vanadium in foods is found in an organic form. Vanadium in food is safer than non-food forms and also appears to be about 50% more effective [39].

Zinc

Most researchers acknowledge that organic zinc is better absorbed than inorganic zinc [71]. Zinc itself is generally found in the human body in ionic form [71,76]; it is often bound with albumin [23,76] or alpha2-macroglobulin [23] or exists as part of one of the many zinc metalloenzymes [23,76]. Zinc is predominantly found in foods as zinc peptide complex (such as that complexed with superoxide dismutase). Zinc is not naturally found in the body as zinc gluconate, zinc orotate, zinc sulfate, nor zinc picolinate. In humans "zinc deficiency does not exist without deficiency of other nutrients" [76].

Zinc deficiency in humans can cause alopecia, impotence, skin problems, immune deficiencies, night blindness, impaired taste, delayed wound healing, impaired appetite, photophobia, difficulty in dark adaptation, growth retardation, and male infertility [23]. Zinc in yeast-containing foods is better absorbed and is a better form for humans than inorganic forms [40,41]. Studies indicate that Food zinc appears to be 1.72-1.75 times more absorbed in the blood than zinc sulfate (1.71 times more than zinc chelate; 6.46 times more than zinc gluconate; 3.11 times more than zinc orotate) and 1.75-1.87 times more retained in the liver than zinc sulfate (1.45 times more than zinc amino acid chelate; 3.68 times more than zinc gluconate; 1.50 times more than zinc orotate) [45,46,51].

Food and Food Processing

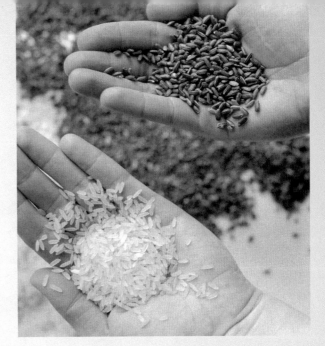

"In the historic struggle for food, humans ate primarily whole foods or so-called natural foods, which underwent little processing... The nutrient content of food usually decreases when it is processed" [77]. "Intensive animal rearing, manipulation of crop production and food processing have altered the qualitative and quantitative balance of nutrients of food consumed by Western society. This change, to which the physiology and biochemistry of man may not be presently adapted is thought to be responsible for the chronic diseases that are rampant in the Industrialized Western Countries" [78]. Some reports suggest that simply taking a synthetic multi-vitamin/mineral formula does not change this [79,80].

Commercial food processing definitely reduces the nutrient content of food [81, 82] and can be dangerous to human health [83]. The refining of whole grains (including wheat, rice, and corn) has resulted in a dramatic reduction of their natural food complex nutrition [11,82]; specifically the milling of wheat to white flour reduces the natural food complex vitamin and mineral content by 40-60% [82]. Food refining appears to reduce trace minerals such as manganese, zinc, and chromium [2] and various macrominerals (such as magnesium) as well [10,56]. The treatment of canned or frozen vegetables with ethylenediaminetetraacetic acid (EDTA) can strip much of the zinc from foods [11]. The high incidences of disorders of calcium metabolism [28] suggest that the forms of calcium being consumed simply do not agree with the body (and sometimes result in calcium loss [11]).

Organically-grown produce appears to contain higher levels of some essential minerals than does conventionally (non-organically) grown produce [84,85] and appears to contain lower levels of toxic heavy metals [86]. Even if modern food practices did not affect nutrition (which they do), all minerals that humans need for optimal health do not exist uniformly in soils. "Soils in many areas of the world are deficient in certain minerals; this can result in low concentrations of major or trace minerals in drinking water, plant crops, and even tissues of farm animals, thus contributing to marginal or deficient dietary intakes of humans [76].

From a geological perspective, a few examples include iodine, molybdenum, cobalt, selenium, and boron [2,70,77]. Although humans need at least twenty minerals (over sixty have been found in the body), most plants can be grown with only the addition of nitrogen, phosphorus, and potassium compounds [2]. If other minerals necessary for human health are reduced in the soil, the plant can (and will) grow without them. This means, though, that constantly farming the same ground can result in the reduction of some of the essential minerals we as humans require for optimal health [78].

Ground Up Rocks Pose Risks

Rock minerals are not optimal for human health and post health risks. Perhaps it should be mentioned that typical multi-vitamin-mineral formulas are dangerous and do not result in optimal health. A study involving 38,772 women in the USA who took synthetic multi-vitamins with ground up rock minerals found that the women died earlier than those who did not take them [87]. Other studies have concluded that the acid-processed rocks that many take as calcium supplements increase risk of cardiovascular disease and other problems [88]—yet those studies did not find problems with food calcium.

Ground-up rocks are dangerous for humans to ingest. Yet, real foods and 100% food vitamins and minerals are beneficial as well as essential to human health and longevity.

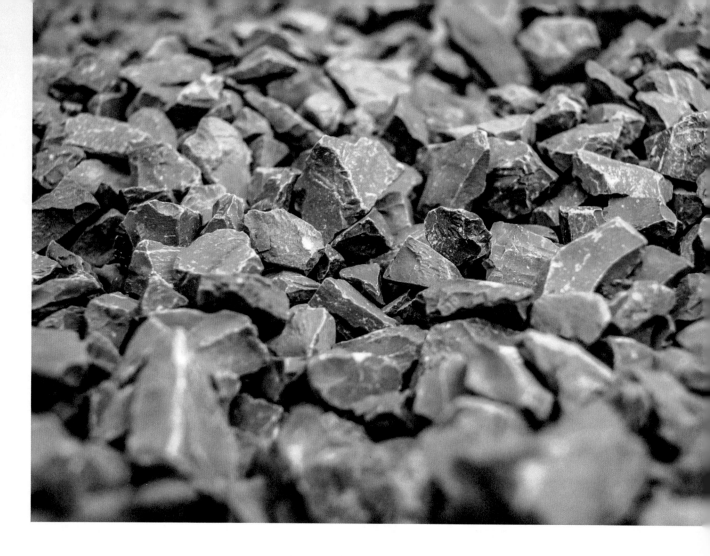

Conclusion

No matter how many industrially produced mineral supplements one takes orally, they will:

1) Never be a truly complete nutrient source.

2) Never replace all the functions of food minerals.

3) Always be unnatural substances to the body.

4) Always strain the body by requiring that it detoxify or somehow dispose of their unnatural structures/chemicals.

5) Never be utilized, absorbed, and retained the same as food nutrients.

6) Not be able to prevent advanced protein glycation end-product formation the same as food nutrients.

7) Never be able to have the antioxidant effects the same as food nutrients.

8) Always be industrial products.

9) Always be composed of petroleum-derivatives, hydrogenated sugars, acids, and/or industrially-processed rocks.

10) Never build optimal health the same as food nutrients.

Industrially processed minerals can have some positive nutritional effects, yet they are not food for humans. Unlike humans, plants have roots or hyphae which aid in the absorption of minerals. Plants actually have the ability to decrease the toxicity of compounds by changing their biochemical forms [14]. Plants are naturally intended to ingest rocks; humans are not [1].

The truth is that plants, or supplements only made from plants, are the best form of mineral supplement for humans, yet most people who take nutritional mineral support consume some type of industrially processed rock.

References

[1] Cronquist A. Plantae. In Synopsis and Classification of Living Organisms, Vol 1. McGraw-Hill, NY, 1982:57

[2] Schroeder HA. The Trace Elements and Man. Devin-Adair, New Greenwich (CT), 1973

[3] Howell E. Enzyme Nutrition. Avery Publishing, Wayne (NJ), 1985

[4] Milne L, Milne M. The Arena of Life: The Dynamics of Ecology. Natural History Press, Garden City (NJ), 1972

[5] Wallace RA. Biology: The World of Life, 6th ed. Harper Collins, New York, 1992

[6] Dietary guidelines in The Weston A. Price Foundation brochure. Weston A. Price Foundation, Washington, 1999

[7] Gehman JM. From the Office of the President: Pseudo-Group Once Again Misleading the Naturopathic Field. Official Bulletin ANA, January 25, 1948:7-8

[8] Shapes SA, Schlussel YR, Cifuentes M. Drug-Nutrient Interactions That Affect Mineral Status. In Handbook of Drug-Nutrient Interactions. Humana Press, Totowa (NJ), 2004: 301-328

[9] Nielsen F. Ultratrace Minerals. In Modern Nutrition in Health and Disease, 8th ed. Lea & Febiger, Phil.,1994:269-286

[10] Turnland JR. Copper. In Modern Nutrition in Health and Disease, 8th ed. Lea & Febiger, Phil.,1994:231-241

[11] Whitney EN, Hamilton EMN. Understanding Nutrition, 4ed. West Publishing, New York, 1987

[12] Beers MH, Berkow R, eds. The Merck Manual of Diagnosis and Therapy, 17th ed. Merck Research Laboratories, Whitehouse Station (NJ), 1999

[13] Thiel RJ. Mineral salts are for plants, food complexed minerals are for humans. ANMA Monitor 1999;3(2):5-10

[14] Huang Y, Chen Y, Tao S. Effect of rhizospheric environment of VA-mycorrhizal plants on forms of Cu, Zn, PB and Cd in polluted soil. Ying Yong Sheng Tai Xye Bao 2000;11(3):431-434

[15] Budvari S, et al eds. The Merck Index, An Encyclopedia of Chemicals, Drugs, and Biologicals, 12th ed. Merck Research Laboratories, Whitehouse Station (NJ), 1996

[16] Anagisawa KY, Rendon-Angeles JC, Shizawa NI, Ishi SO. Topotaxial replacement of chlorapatite by hydroxy during hydrothermal ion exchange. Am Mineralogist 1999;84:1861-1869

[17] DiTomaso JM. Yellow starthistle: chemical control. Proceedings of the CalEPPC Symposium, 1996, as updated 5/2/02

[18] Vitamin-Mineral Manufacturing Guide Nutrient Empowerment, volume 1. Nutrition Resource, Lakeport (CA), 1986

[19] Hojo Y, Hashimoto I, Miyamoto Y, Kawazoe S, Mizutani T. In vivo toxicity and glutathione, ascorbic acid, and copper level changes induced in mouse liver and kidney by copper (II) gluconate, a nutrient supplement. Yakugaku Zasshi 2000;120(3):311-314

[20] City of Lubbock. www.solidwaste.ci.lubbock.tx.us/hhw/hhw.htm 7/18/02
Cunnane SC. Zinc: Clinical and Biochemical Significance. CRC Press, Boca Raton (FL),1988

[21] Patrick J. What most people don't know about vitamin C. The Alacer Health Report, Foothill Ranch (CA), 1994

[22] Jensen B. The Chemistry of Man. Bernard Jensen, Escondido (CA),1983

[23] King JC, Keen CL. Zinc. In Modern Nutrition in Health and Disease, 9th ed. Williams & Wilkins, Balt., 1999:223-239

[24] Chromium picolinate, rev. 6/96B.BLI website, July 16, 2002

[25] Implications of the 'other half' of a mineral compound. Albion Research Notes 2000;9(3):1-5

[26] Stoecker B.J. Chromium. In Modern Nutrition in Health and Disease, 10th ed. Lippincott Williams & Wilkins, Phil., 2005: 332-337

[27] Turnland JR. Bioavailability of dietary minerals to humans: the stable isotope approach. Crit Rev Food Sci Nutr 1991;30(4);387-396

[28] Schumann K, et al. Bioavailability of oral vitamins, minerals, and trace minerals in perspective. Arzneimittelforshcung 1997;47(4):369-380

[29] El-Bayoumy K, Richie JP Jr, Boyiri T, Komninou D, Prokopczyk B, Trushin N, Kleinman W, Cox J, Pittman B, Colosimo S. Influence of Selenium-Enriched Yeast Supplementation on Biomarkers of Oxidative Damage and Hormone Status in Healthy Adult Males: A Clinical Pilot Study. Cancer Epidemiol Biomarkers Prev. 2002;11:1459-1465

[30] Hamet P, et al. The evaluation of the scientific evidence for a relationship between calcium and hypertension. J Nutr, 1995;125:311S-400S

[31] Ensminger AH, Ensminger ME, Konlade JE, Robson JRK. Food & Nutrition Encyclopedia, 2nd ed. CRC Press, New York, 1993

[32] Avery SV, Howlett NG, Radice S. Copper toxicity towards Saccharomyces cerevisiae: dependence on plasma fatty acid composition. Appl Environ Microbiol 1996;62(11):3960-3966

[33] Wi'snicka R, Krzepiko A, Krawiec Z, Bili'nski T. Protective role of superoxide dismutase in iron toxicity in yeast. Biochem Mol Biol Int 1998;44(3):635-641

[34] Wood R.J., Ronnenberg A.G. Iron. In Modern Nutrition in Health and Disease, 10th ed. Lippincott William & Wilkins, Phil, 2006: 248-270

[35] Rude R.K., Shils M.E. Magnesium. In Modern Nutrition in Health and Disease, 10th ed. Lippincott William & Wilkins, Phil, 2006: 223-247

[36] Buchman A. Manganese. In Modern Nutrition in Health & Disease, 10th ed. Lippincott William & Wilkins, Phil, 2006:326-331

[37] Beloosesky Y, Grinblat J, Weiss A, Grosman B, Gafter U, Chagnac A. Electrolyte disorders following oral sodium phosphate administration for bowel cleansing in elderly patients. Arch Intern Med. 2003;163(7):803-808

[38] Biotechnology in the Feed Industry. Nottingham Press, UK, 1995: 257-267

[39] Badmaev V, Prakash S, Majeed M. Vanadium: a review of its potential role in the fight against diabetes. J Altern Complement Med. 1999;5(3):273-291

[40] Andlid TA, Veide J, Sandberg AS. Metabolism of extracellular inositol hexaphosphate (phytate) by Saccharomyces cerevisiae. Int J. Food Microbiology. 2004;97(2):157-169

[41] King JC, Cousins RJ. Zinc. In Modern Nutrition in Health and Disease, 10th ed. Lipponcott Williams & Wilkins, Phil., 2005:271-285

[42] Thiel R, Fowkes S. Can cognitive deterioration associated with Down syndrome be reduced? Med Hypo, 2005; 64(3):524-532

[43] Jenkins DJA, Wolever TMS, and Jenkins AL. Diet Factors Affecting Nutrient Absorption and Metabolism. In Modern Nutrition in Health and Disease, 8th ed. Lea and Febiger, Phil.:583-602, 1994

[44] Vinson, J.A., Jennifer M. Stella, J.M., Flanagan, T.J. Selenium yeast is an effective in vitro and in vivo antioxidant and hypolipemic agent in normal hamsters. Nutritional Research, 1998, Vol 18, No. 4: 735-742

[45] Vinson J, Bose P, Lemoine L, Hsiao KH. Bioavailability studies. In Nutrient Availability: Chemical and Biological Aspects. Royal Society of Chemistry, Cambridge (UK) 1989:125-127

[46] Vinson JA, Bose P. Comparison of bio-availability of trace elements in inorganic salts, amino acid chelates, and yeast. Mineral Elements 80, Proceedings II, Helsinki, Dec 9-11, 1981

[47] Vinson J, Mazur T, Bose P. Comparisons of different forms of calcium on blood pressure of normotensive males. Nutr Reports Intl, 1987;36(3):497-505

[48] Vinson JA, Hsiao, KH. Comparative effect of various forms of chromium on serum glucose: an assay for biologically active chromium. Nutr Reports Intl,1985;32(1):1-7

[49] Vinson JA, Bose P. The effect of high chromium yeast on the blood glucose control and blood lipids of normal and diabetic human subjects. Nutr Reports Intl, 1984;30(4):911-918

[50] Vinson JA, Howard TB. Inhibition of protein glycation and advanced glycation end products by ascorbic acid and other vitamins and nutrients. Nutr Biochemistry, 1996;7:659-663

[51] Vinson J. Rat zinc bioavailability study. University of Scranton, Scranton (PA), 1991

[52] Vinson J. Bioavailability of magnesium. University of Scranton, Scranton (PA), 1991

[53] Frequently Asked Questions. www.albionlabs.com July 19, 2002

[54] Rouhi AM. Escorting metal ions: protein chaperone protects, guides, copper ions in transit. Chem Eng News 1999;11:34-35

[55] Himelblau E, et al. Identification of a functional homolog of the yeast copper homeostasis gene ATX1 from Arabidopsis. Plant Physiol 1998;117(4):1227-1234

[56] Lapinskas PJ, Lin SJ, Culotta VC. The role of Saccharomyces cerevisiae CCC1 gene in the homeostasis of manganese ions. Mol Microbiol 1996;21(3):519-528

[57] Allen LH, Wood RJ. Calcium and Phosphorus. In Modern Nutrition in Health and Disease, 8th ed. Lea & Febiger, Phil.,1994:144-163

[58] Heaney RP, Dowell MS, Barger-Lux MJ. Absorption of calcium as the carbonate and citrate salts, with some observations on method. Osteoporosis Int, 1999;9:19-23

[59] Timon S. Mineral Logic: Understanding the Mineral Transportsport System. Advanced Nutrition Research: Ellicottville (NY),1985

[60] Burger S. Vitamins and Minerals for Health. Wild Rose College of Natural Healing, Calgary,1988

[61] Orlov SN, Li JM, Tremblay J, Hamet P. Genes of intracellular calcium metabolism and blood pressure control in primary hypertension. Semin Nephrol. 1995 Nov;15(6):569-592

[62] Osborne G, et al. Evidence for the relationship of calcium to blood pressure. Nutr Reviews, 1996;54(12):365-381

[63] Yamamoto ME., et al. Lack of blood pressure effect with calcium and magnesium supplementation with adults with high-normal blood pressure results from phase I of the Trials of Hypertension and Prevention (TOHP). Ann Epidem, 1995;5:96-107

[64] Afghani A, Johnson CA. Resting blood pressure and bone mineral content are inversely related in overweight and obese Hispanic women. Am J Hypertens. 2006;19(3):286-292

[65] Knight KB, Keith RE. Effects of oral calcium supplementation via calcium carbonate versus diet on blood pressure and serum calcium in young, normotensive adults. J Opt Nutr, 1994;3(4):152-158

[66] Weaver CM, Heaney R. Calcium. In Modern Nutrition in Health & Disease, 10th ed. Lippincott Williams & Wilkins, Phil., 2006:194-210

[67] Nielson F. Chromium. In Modern Nutrition in Health and Disease, 8th ed. Lea & Febiger, Phil.,1994:264-268

[68] Hendlor S, Rorvik D, eds. PDR for Nutritional Supplements, 1st ed. Medical Economics, Montvale (NJ), 2001

[69] Turnland JR. Copper. In Modern Nutrition in Health and Disease, 8th ed. Lea & Febiger, Phil.,1994:231-241

[70] Hetzel BS, Clugston GA. Iodine. In Modern Nutrition in Health and Disease, 9th ed. Lea & Febiger, Phil.,1999:253-264

[71] Greene HL and Moran JR. The Gastrointestinal Tract: Regulation of Nutrient Absorption. In Modern Nutrition in Health and Disease, 8th ed. Lea and Febiger, Phil.,1994:549-568

[72] Fairbanks VF. Iron in Medicine and Nutrition. In Modern Nutrition in Health and Disease, 8th ed. Lea & Febiger, Phil.,1994:185-213

[73] Shils M. Magnesium. In Modern Nutrition in Health and Disease, 8th ed. Lea & Febiger, Phil.,1994:164-184

[74] Levander OA, Burk RF. Selenium. In Modern Nutrition in Health and Disease, 8th ed. Lea & Febiger, Phil.,1994:242-263

[75] Whitaker J. Minerals, part 1: Cut your cancer risk with selenium. Health & Healing, 1999;9(4):6-8

[76] Cunnane SC. Zinc: Clinical and Biochemical Significance. CRC Press, Boca Raton (FL),1988

[77] Bauernfeind JC. Nutrification of foods. In Modern Nutrition in Health and Disease, 8th ed. Lea & Febiger, Phil.,1994:1579-1592

[78] Ghebremeskel K, Crawford MA. Nutrition and health in relation to food production and processing. Nutr Health, 1994;9(4):237-253

[79] Bazzarre TL, Hopkins RG, Wu SM, Murdoch SD. Chronic disease risk factors in vitamin/mineral supplement users and nonusers in a farm population. J Am Coll Nutr, 1991;10(3):247-257

[80] Sax NI, Lewis RJ. Hawley's Condensed Chemical Dictionary, 11th ed. Van Nostrand Rheinhold, New York,1987

[81] Burr-Madsen A. Gateways College of Natural Therapies, Module 1. Gateway College, Shingle Springs (CA), 1996

[82] Erdman JW, Poneros-Schneir AG. Factors affecting the nutritive value in processed foods. In Modern Nutrition in Health and Disease, 8th ed. Lea & Febiger, Phil.,1994:1569-1578

[83] Ascherio A and Willett WC. Health effects of trans fatty acids. Am J Clin Nutr, 1997;66:1006S-1010S

[84] Hornick SB. Factors affecting the nutritional quality of crops. AM J Alternative Ag,1992;7(1-2)

[85] Barański M, et al. Higher antioxidant and lower cadmium concentrations and lower incidence of pesticide residues in organically grown crops: a systematic literature review and meta-analyses. Br J Nutr. 2014 Jun 26:1-18.

[86] Smith BL. Organic foods vs. supermarket foods: J Applied Nutr,1993;45(1):35-39

87] Mursu J., et al. Dietary Supplements and Mortality Rate in Older WomenThe Iowa Women's Health Study. Arch Intern Med. 2011;171(18):1625-1633

[88] Boland MJ, et al. Calcium Supplements and Cardiovascular Risk. Ther Adv in Drug Safe. 2013;4(5):199-210

ARE YOUR SUPPLEMENTS 100% FOOD OR ROCKS?

If you and your clients are like most health-conscious Americans today, you have serious concerns about the quality of our food supply (Genetically Modified Organisms, preservatives, chemical additives, commercial processing), enough so, that you are taking a multiple vitamin and mineral supplement. Shouldn't those supplemental nutrients be from Food?

Sadly, most supplement formulas sold today do not contain vitamins and minerals as found in foods. Even though the label often claims that the product is "natural", the ingredients are almost always USP synthetic vitamins and commercially mined and processed rocks. These rocks are altered using industrial chemicals, such as gluconic acid (which is used in cleaning compounds), to form isolated rock salts, and while rocks are natural food for plants, they are not a natural food for humans.

Nature intended that plants would ingest rocks and in turn, humans would eat the plants. Plants have the ability to change the chemical compounds found in rocks and to detoxify them. Plants ingest rocks, humans eat plants. This is called the "Food Chain".

Commercially processed rocks are used in the manufacturing of supplements because they are much cheaper to produce than the nutrients found in Food Research Food supplements.

Food Vitamins and Minerals are made from natural food nutrients…

Compare these electron microscope photographs (same magnification), and you'll see the difference between the Food nutrients on the left, and isolated U.S.P. synthetic vitamins and mineral salts on the right. Food nutrients do not even look the same as U.S.P. vitamins and mineral salts. Not only do most of the nutrients differ in their physical appearance, they differ chemically and structurally as well.

Food nutrients tend to have a more rounded appearance, whereas U.S.P. vitamins have a more crystalline or rock-like appearance, as do most mineral salts used to produce synthetic supplements.

STOP the USE of SYNTHETIC VITAMINS

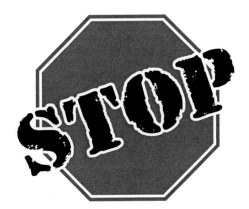

Eating Industrial Chemicals!

FOOD VITAMINS & MINERALS	NON-FOOD VITAMINS & MINERALS
Food Vitamin B-1	*Thiamin HCL*
Food Vitamin C	*Ascorbic Acid*
Food Zinc	*Zinc Chloride*

CHIRO NUTRITION CHART™

Vertebrae	Chiropractic Connection	Product Considerations
Cervical 1	Blood supply to head, pituitary	Inflam-Enzymes (4), Serious Brain Enhancer (3), Hematic Formula (1)
Cervical 2	Eyes, optic nerve forehead	Inflam-Enzymes (4), Complete Eye Health (1)
Cervical 3	Cheeks, teeth, trifacial nerve	Inflam-Enzymes (6), Cal-Mag Complex (2)
Cervical 4	Nose, lips, mouth	Inflam-Enzymes (6), Complete Smell & Taste (3)
Cervical 5	Vocal cords, neck glands	Inflam-Enzymes (4), Advanced Joint Complex (3)
Cervical 6	Neck muscles, shoulders	Inflam-Enzymes (6), Magnesium Complex (3)
Cervical 7	Thyroid gland	Inflam-Enzymes (4), Metabolic Thyro (3)
Thoracic 1	Hands, trachea	Inflam-Enzymes (6), Advanced Joint Complex (3)
Thoracic 2	Heart, including its valves	Inflam-Enzymes (4), Cardio-Power (3), Omega 3/EPA/DHA (2)
Thoracic 3	Lungs, bronchials, breasts	Inflam-Enzymes (4), Simply Lung (2) or Simply Mammary (2)
Thoracic 4	Gall bladder, bile duct	Inflam-Enzymes (4), GB Support (3)
Thoracic 5	Liver, blood	Inflam-Enzymes (4), Liva-Detox & Support (3), Hematic Formula (1)
Thoracic 6	Stomach	Inflam-Enzymes (4), Digesti-Pan (3-6)
Thoracic 7	Pancreas	Inflam-Enzymes (4), Simply Pancreas (3)
Thoracic 8	Spleen, diaphragm	Inflam-Enzymes (4), Simply Spleen (3)
Thoracic 9	Adrenal glands	Inflam-Enzymes (4), Simply Adrenal (3) or Anxie-Tone (3)
Thoracic 10	Kidneys	Inflam-Enzymes (4), Uro-Kid Support (3-6)
Thoracic 11	Kidneys, ureters	Inflam-Enzymes (4), Uro-Kid Support (3-6) or Arginase Bladder (3-6)
Thoracic 12	Small intestines, lymph nodes	Inflam-Enzymes (4), Digesti-Pan (3-6) or Simply Pancreas (3-6)
Lumbar 1	Large intestines	Inflam-Enzymes (6), Para-Dysbio-Zyme (4) or GB Support (3)
Lumbar 2	Abdomen	Inflam-Enzymes (6), Digesti-Pan (3-6)
Lumbar 3	Sex organs	Inflam-Enzymes (4), Feminine Advantage (3) or Prosta-Power (3)
Lumbar 4	Prostate, lower back muscles	Inflam-Enzymes (6), Prosta-Power (3) or Magnesium Complex (4)
Lumbar 5	Lower legs, feet, toes	Inflam-Enzymes (6), Cal-Mag Complex (2) or Vegetarian Adrenal (2)
Sacrum	Hips, buttocks	Inflam-Enzymes (4), Advanced Joint Complex (4)
Coccyx	Rectum, anus	Inflam-Enzymes (4), Para-Dysbio-Zyme (6)

Other Concerns	Chiropractic Connection	Product Considerations
Ankles	Ankles	Uro-Kid Support (4) or Advanced Joint Complex (3)
Bones	Bones	Calcium Complex (4), D Complex (1) or Cal-Mag Complex (3)
Elbows	Elbow	Inflam-Enzymes (6), Advanced Joint Complex (2)
Health	All systems	Vitamin-Mineral (1-2)
Injury	Joint, muscle	Inflam-Enzymes (8), Omega 3/EPA/DHA (4)
Knee	Knee	Advanced Joint Complex (3-6), also avoid caffeine
Moving aches	Muscles, joints	Inflam-Enzymes (6), Migratrol (3)
Muscles	Muscles	Magnesium Complex (3), Omega 3/EPA/DHA (4)
Wrists	Wrists	Inflam-Enzymes (6), Vitamin B-6, B-12, & Folate (2)

Note: Many spinal nerves are connected to multiple organs/systems, thus this chart is not always applicable. The above chart also normally is not including suggestions when a problem is caused by some type of infection. The amount of tablets/capsules often taken per day is shown between the (). None of these statements have been approved by the US Food and Drug Administration, Health Canada, or similar authorities.

Made in the USA
Middletown, DE
11 September 2024

60771848R10073